U0235557

第 **3** 版

实用人体解剖
彩色图谱

主　编　羊惠君

副主编　周鸿鹰　李　华

编　委（按姓氏笔画排序）

　　　　冯　轼　　朱　磊　　刘少文

　　　　刘蜀生　　羊惠君　　李　华

　　　　汪贵明　　周鸿鹰　　赵志伟

　　　　姜德建　　曹　霞　　廖世华

PRACTICAL
COLORED ATLAS
OF
HUMAN ANATOMY

人民卫生出版社

图书在版编目（CIP）数据

实用人体解剖彩色图谱/羊惠君主编. —3 版. —北京：
人民卫生出版社,2017

ISBN 978-7-117-25811-1

Ⅰ.①实… Ⅱ.①羊… Ⅲ.①人体解剖学-图谱
Ⅳ.①R322-64

中国版本图书馆 CIP 数据核字（2017）第 326616 号

| 人卫智网 | www. ipmph. com | 医学教育、学术、考试、健康，购书智慧智能综合服务平台 |
| 人卫官网 | www. pmph. com | 人卫官方资讯发布平台 |

版权所有,侵权必究!

实用人体解剖彩色图谱
第 3 版

主　　编：羊惠君
出版发行：人民卫生出版社（中继线 010-59780011）
地　　址：北京市朝阳区潘家园南里 19 号
邮　　编：100021
E－mail：pmph @ pmph. com
购书热线：010-59787592　010-59787584　010-65264830
印　　刷：北京人卫印刷厂
经　　销：新华书店
开　　本：787×1092　1/16　　印张：19
字　　数：462 千字
版　　次：2001 年 1 月第 1 版　　2018 年 3 月第 3 版
　　　　　2018 年 3 月第 3 版第 1 次印刷（总第 16 次印刷）
标准书号：ISBN 978-7-117-25811-1/R·25812
定　　价：98.00 元

打击盗版举报电话：010-59787491　E-mail：WQ @ pmph. com
（凡属印装质量问题请与本社市场营销中心联系退换）

第 3 版前言

自 2001 年《实用人体解剖彩色图谱》和《简明人体解剖彩色图谱》相继出版以来已有 16 个年头。这两本图谱得益于大量精致的人体实物标本,真实地显示结构器官的形态、质地、位置和毗邻关系,一直以来是医学生、研究生学习人体解剖学知识普遍使用的参考书,也得到解剖界同行和临床医务工作者积极的反馈。

根据使用者的意见和建议,2015 年我们完成了《实用人体解剖彩色图谱》第 2 版。该版增加了一些新制作的较大型实物标本照片,将《简明人体解剖彩色图谱》的部分插图编排在其中,丰富了这本图谱的内容,并逐一仔细校对了该版图谱中所有标注结构的解剖学名词。

《实用人体解剖彩色图谱》第 3 版保持了第 2 版的内容,仍按人体局部划分为下肢、上肢、胸、腹、盆和会阴、背和头颈 7 个局部章节,"绪论"为首个章节,"中枢神经系统"为最后的单一章节。

借第 3 版前言,我们衷心感谢人民卫生出版社领导和专家团队。他们对《实用人体解剖彩色图谱》的出版及修订非常关心和支持。各位专家利用其丰富的专业知识对图谱的策划、编写进行了悉心的指导,并对图谱的编辑、版式、照片调色做了大量的具体工作。同时,我们也非常感谢曾给我们提出非常有价值意见和建议的同行和读者,你们的意见和建议使我们受益匪浅。

虽然我们在编写过程中竭尽全力,但因水平所限,不妥之处和错误在所难免,敬请广大读者和解剖界同仁不吝赐教。

编 者
2018 年 2 月于成都

使用说明

　　全书对人体解剖学实验室 381 件精心制作的实物标本拍摄了彩色照片 452 张,绘制解剖结构示意图 22 幅,还有活体解剖结构彩色照片 4 张,牙齿的 X 线片 1 张,共计编排图号 347 个。

　　本图谱主要按照人体局部划分章节,分为下肢、上肢、胸、腹、盆与会阴、背、头与颈 7 个局部章节,以及全身各大系统概论和独立的中枢神经系统 2 个章节,共 9 个章节。

　　每个局部章节先安排骨和关节的内容。然后依分区、由浅到深的层次,安排肌、神经、血管和器官的内容。这本彩色图谱为读者呈现了人体解剖结构真实的形状、颜色、大小、位置和与其他结构的毗邻关系,还可同时看到器官的神经支配和血液供应,逼真地显示了人体解剖结构较为全面的知识。此外,还有部分结构变异的情况、断层解剖图以及铸型标本图。这些都是能在实验室解剖出来、能观察到的,方便临床医学专业、口腔医学专业及相关专业学生进行医学专业训练时使用,也可作为临床医师实践的参考。

　　为方便读者使用,本图谱在每个图题中说明结构显示的方位。采用引线和阿拉伯数字在图上标注结构,在图旁同时介绍结构的中英文解剖学名词。并且,本图谱后附有以汉语拼音为序的中英文解剖学名词索引。读者使用时可按目录以局部和图号查找某一结构,也可按汉语拼音先在索引中查找结构名词,并根据索引中标出的页码找到该结构。

目 录
CONTENTS

目录 **CONTENTS**

8

目录 **CONTENTS**

10

第 7 章　背　Chapter 7　Back ·························· 151（—161）

第 8 章　头与颈　Chapter 8　Head and Neck ············· 162（—218）

目录 **CONTENTS**

16

第 9 章　中枢神经系统　Chapter 9　Central Nervous System　··· 219（—248）

第 1 章　绪 论

Chapter 1　Introduction

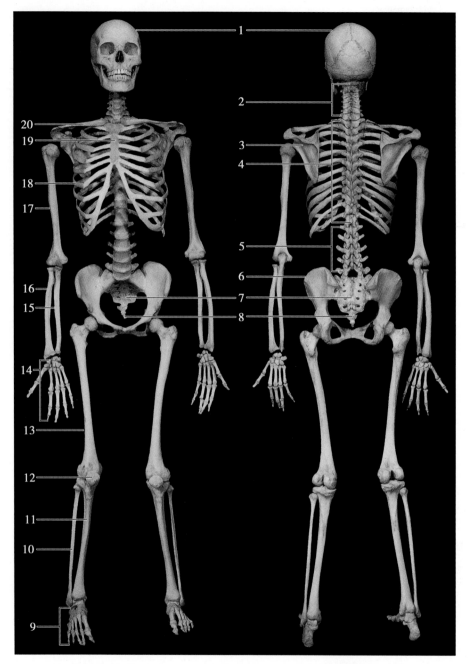

A. 前面观 Anterior view　　　　　B. 后面观 Posterior view

图 1-1　全身骨骼 Skeleton of human body

1. 颅 cranium(skull)
2. 颈椎 cervical vertebrae
3. 肩胛骨 scapula
4. 胸椎 thoracic vertebrae
5. 腰椎 lumbar vertcbrae
6. 髋骨 hip bone
7. 骶骨 sacrum

8. 尾骨 coccyx
9. 足骨 bones of foot
10. 腓骨 fibula
11. 胫骨 tibia
12. 髌骨 patella
13. 股骨 femur
14. 手骨 bones of hand

15. 尺骨 ulna
16. 桡骨 radius
17. 肱骨 humerus
18. 肋 ribs
19. 胸骨 sternum
20. 锁骨 clavicle

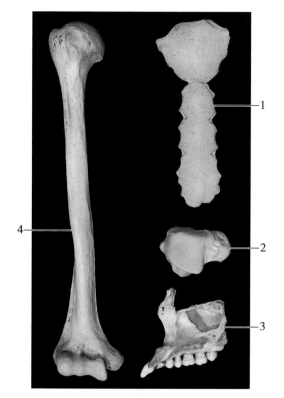

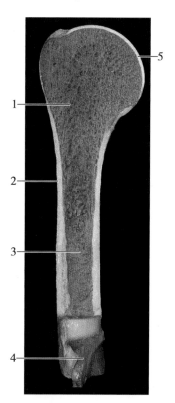

图 1-2 骨的形态 Shape of bones
1. 扁骨 flat bone
2. 短骨 short bone
3. 不规则骨 irregular bone
4. 长骨 long bone

图 1-3 骨的构造(股骨上端剖面)
Structure of bone(section of upper part of femur)
1. 松质骨 spongy bone
2. 密质骨 compact bone
3. 骨髓 bone marrow
4. 骨膜 periosteum
5. 关节软骨 articular cartilage

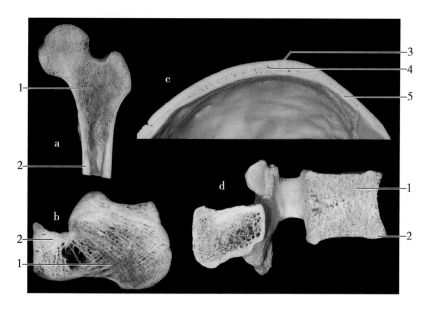

图 1-4 骨的类型
Type of bones
a. 股骨上端剖面 section of upper part of femur
b. 跟骨剖面 section of calcaneus
c. 顶骨剖面 section of parietal bone
d. 椎骨剖面 section of vertebra
1. 松质骨 spongy bone
2. 密质骨 compact bone
3. 外板 outer table
4. 板障 diploë
5. 内板 inner table

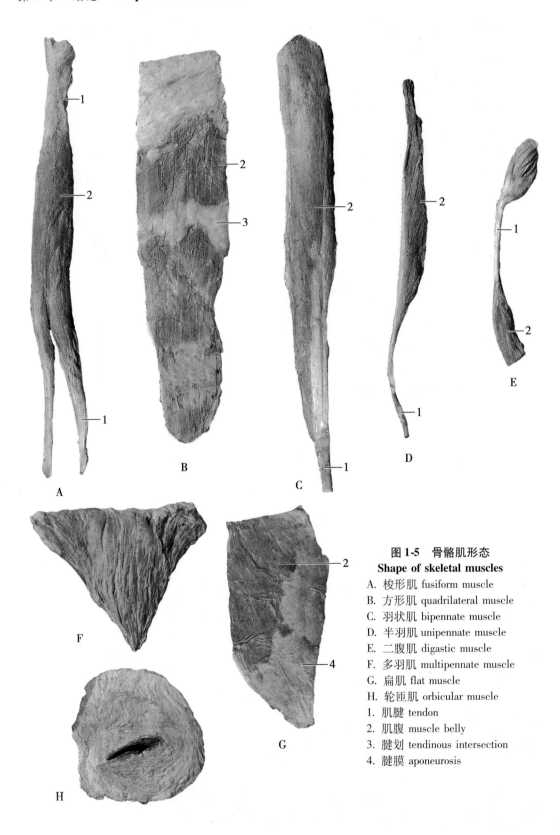

图 1-5　骨骼肌形态
Shape of skeletal muscles
A. 梭形肌 fusiform muscle
B. 方形肌 quadrilateral muscle
C. 羽状肌 bipennate muscle
D. 半羽肌 unipennate muscle
E. 二腹肌 digastic muscle
F. 多羽肌 multipennate muscle
G. 扁肌 flat muscle
H. 轮匝肌 orbicular muscle
1. 肌腱 tendon
2. 肌腹 muscle belly
3. 腱划 tendinous intersection
4. 腱膜 aponeurosis

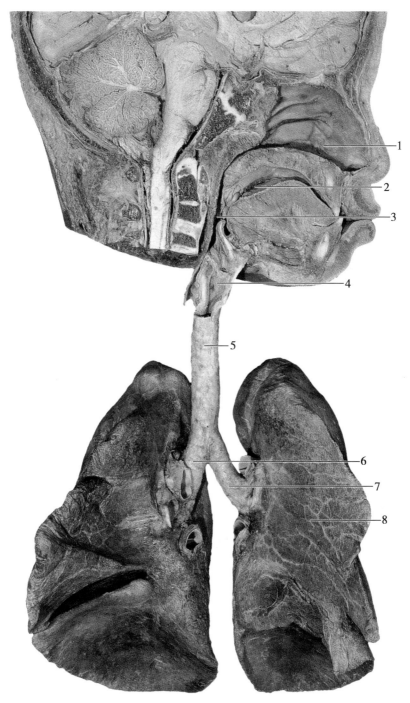

图 1-6 呼吸系统（前面观）Respiratory system（anterior view）

1. 鼻腔 nasal cavity
2. 口腔 oral cavity
3. 咽 pharynx
4. 喉腔 larynx cavity
5. 气管 trachea
6. 右主支气管 right principal bronchus
7. 左主支气管 left principal bronchus
8. 肺 lung

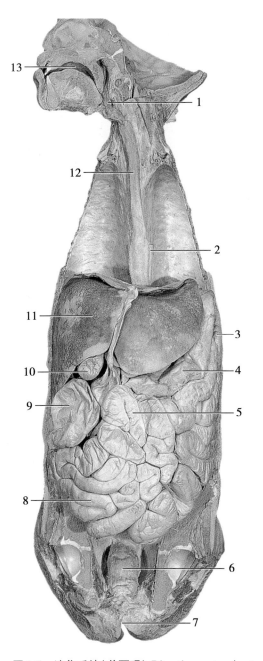

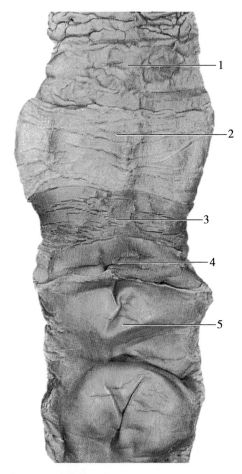

图 1-8　肠壁的层次 Layers of intestinal wall

1. 黏膜 mucosa
2. 黏膜下层 submucosa
3. 内环肌层 internal circular layer of musularis externa
4. 外纵肌层 external longitudinal layer of muscularis externa
5. 外膜(浆膜) adventitia(serosa)

图 1-7　消化系统(前面观) Digestive system(anterior view)

1. 咽 pharynx
2. 胸主动脉 thoracic aorta
3. 脾 spleen
4. 胃 stomach
5. 空肠 jejunum
6. 直肠 rectum
7. 肛门 anus
8. 回肠 ileum
9. 结肠右曲 right colic flexure
10. 胆囊 gallbladder
11. 肝 liver
12. 食管 esophagus
13. 口腔 oral cavity

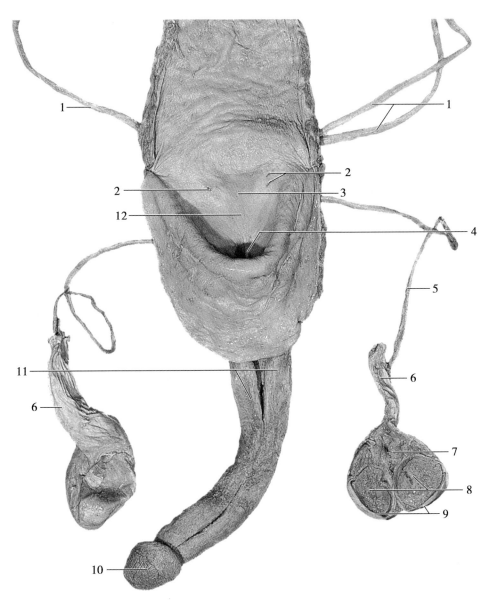

图 1-9 男性膀胱和生殖系统（前面观）
Male urinary bladder and reproductive system（anterior view）

1. 输尿管 ureter（左侧为双输尿管
   duplex ureters appear on left side）
2. 输尿管口 ureteric orifice
3. 输尿管间襞 interureteric fold
4. 尿道内口 internal urethral orifice
5. 输精管 vas deferens
6. 精索 spermatic cord
7. 附睾 epididymis
8. 睾丸 testis
9. 白膜 tunica albuginea
10. 阴茎头 glans of penis
11. 阴茎脚 crus of penis
12. 膀胱三角 trigone of urinary bladder

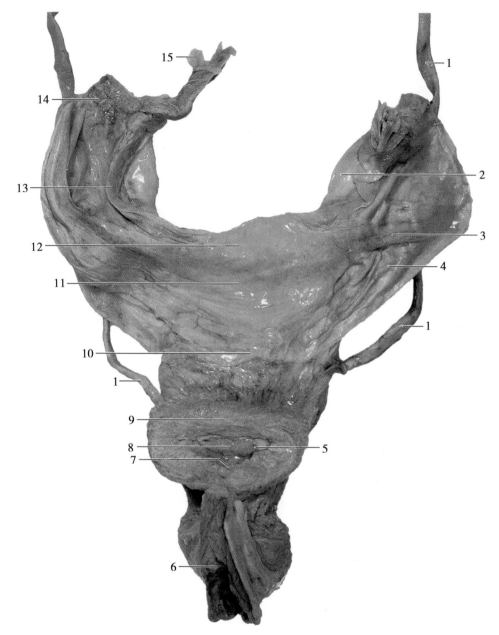

图 1-10　女性生殖系统（前面观）Female reproductive system（anterior view）

1. 输尿管 ureter
2. 卵巢 ovary
3. 子宫圆韧带 round ligament of uterus
4. 子宫阔韧带 broad ligament of uterus
5. 输尿管口 ureteric orifice
6. 女阴 female pudendum
7. 尿道内口 internal urethral orifice
8. 输尿管间襞 interureteric fold
9. 膀胱 urinary bladder
10. 子宫颈 neck of uterus
11. 子宫体 body of uterus
12. 子宫底 fundus of uterus
13. 输卵管 uterine tube
14. 卵巢悬韧带 suspensory ligament of ovary
15. 输卵管伞 fimbriae of uterine tube

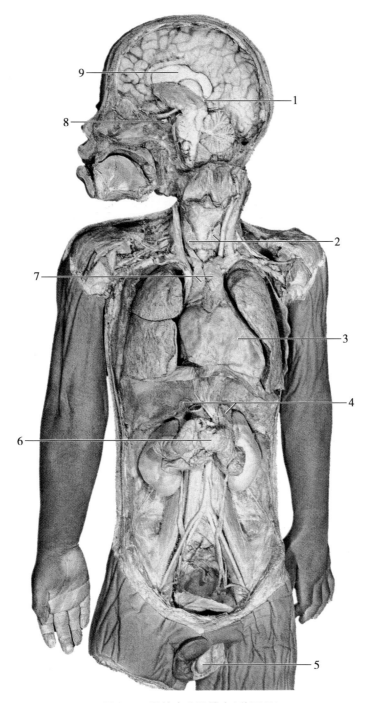

图 1-11　男性内分泌器官（前面观）
Endocrine organs of male（anterior view）

1. 松果体 pineal body
2. 甲状腺 thyroid gland
3. 心包 pericardium
4. 肾上腺 suprarenal gland
5. 睾丸 testis
6. 胰 pancreas
7. 胸腺 thymus
8. 垂体 pituitary gland
9. 胼胝体 corpus callosum

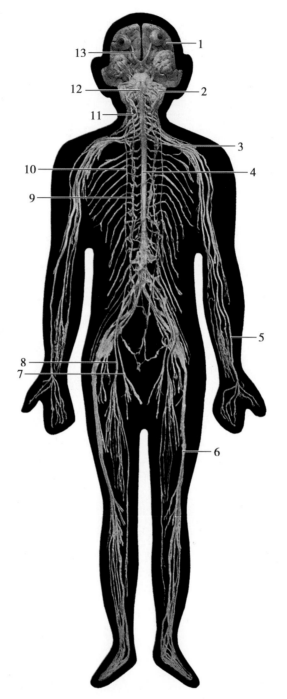

图 1-12　神经系统（前面观）Nervous system（anterior view）

1. 大脑半球 cerebral hemisphere
2. 小脑 cerebellum
3. 臂丛 brachial plexus
4. 脊髓 spinal cord
5. 正中神经 median nerve
6. 坐骨神经 sciatic nerve
7. 闭孔神经 obturator nerve
8. 股神经 femoral nerve
9. 交感干 sympathetic trunk
10. 膈神经 phrenic nerve
11. 迷走神经（Ⅹ）vagus nerve（Ⅹ）
12. 脑干 brain stem
13. 视神经（Ⅱ）optic nerve（Ⅱ）

第 2 章　下肢

Chapter 2　Lower Limb

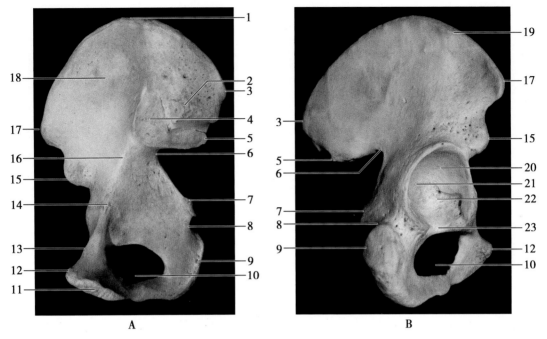

图 2-1　右侧髋骨 Right hip bone

A. 内面观 Internal view　B. 外面观 External view

1. 髂嵴 iliac crest
2. 髂粗隆 iliac tuberosity
3. 髂后上棘 posterior superior iliac spine
4. 耳状面 auricular surface
5. 髂后下棘 posterior inferior iliac spine
6. 坐骨大切迹 greater sciatic notch
7. 坐骨棘 ischial spine
8. 坐骨小切迹 lesser sciatic notch
9. 坐骨结节 ischial tuberosity
10. 闭孔 obturator foramen
11. 耻骨联合面 symphysial surface
12. 耻骨结节 pubic tubercle
13. 耻骨梳 pecten of pubis
14. 髂耻隆起 iliopubic eminence
15. 髂前下棘 anterior inferior iliac spine
16. 弓状线 arcuate line
17. 髂前上棘 anterior superior iliac spine
18. 髂窝 iliac fossa
19. 髂结节 tubercle of iliac crest
20. 髋臼 acetabulum
21. 月状面 lunate surface
22. 髋臼窝 acetabular fossa
23. 髋臼切迹 acetabular notch

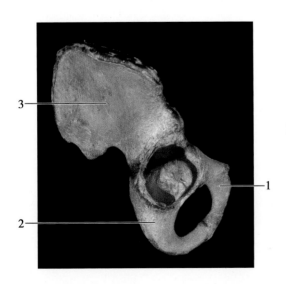

图 2-2　右侧婴儿髋骨（外面观）
Right infant hip bone（external view）

1. 耻骨 pubis
2. 坐骨 ischium
3. 髂骨 ilium

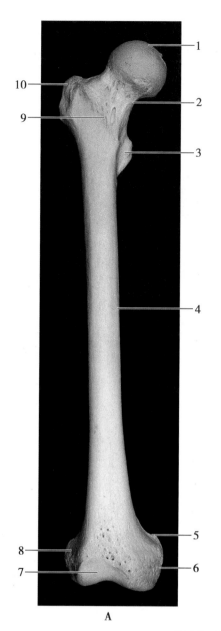

A

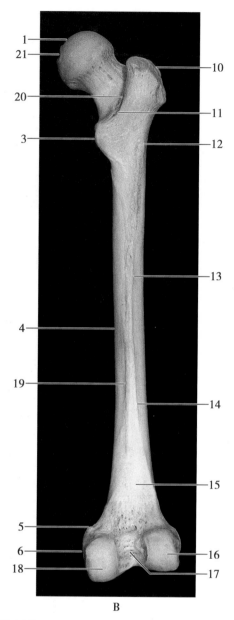

B

图 2-3　右侧股骨 Right femur

A. 前面观 Anterior view　B. 后面观 Posterior view

1. 股骨头 head of femur
2. 股骨颈 neck of femur
3. 股骨小转子 lesser trochanter of femur
4. 股骨体 shaft of femur
5. 收肌结节 adductor tubercle
6. 内上髁 medial epicondyle
7. 髌面 patellar surface
8. 外上髁 lateral epicondyle
9. 转子间线 intertrochanteric line
10. 股骨大转子 greater trochanter of femur
11. 转子间嵴 intertrochanteric crest

12. 臀肌粗隆 gluteal tuberosity
13. 粗线 linea aspera
14. 外侧唇 external lip
15. 腘面 popliteal surface
16. 外侧髁 lateral condyle
17. 髁间窝 intercondylar fossa
18. 内侧髁 medial condyle
19. 内侧唇 internal lip
20. 转子窝 trochanteric fossa
21. 股骨头凹 fovea of femoral head

13

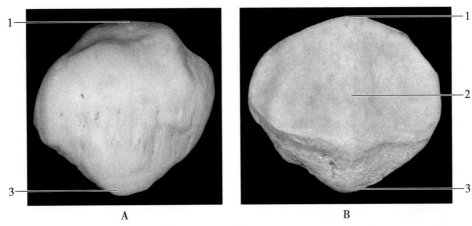

图 2-4 右侧髌骨 Right patella
A. 前面观 Anterior view B. 后面观 Posterior view
1. 髌底 base of patella   3. 髌尖 apex of patella
2. 关节面 articular surface of patella

胫骨 Tibia
A. 右侧骨 Right bone
B. 左侧骨 Left bone
1. 内侧髁 medial condyle
2. 胫骨粗隆 tuberosity of tibia
3. 胫骨体 shaft of tibia
4. 内踝 medial malleolus
5. 内踝关节面 medial malleolar articular surface
6. 下关节面 inferior articular surface
7. 上关节面 superior articular surface
8. 外侧髁 lateral condyle
9. 腓关节面 fibular articular facet
10. 腓切迹 fibular notch
11. 比目鱼肌线 soleal line
12. 髁间隆起 intercondylar eminence

腓骨 Fibula
A. 左侧骨 Left bone
B. 右侧骨 Right bone
1. 腓骨头尖 apex of head of fibula
2. 腓骨头 head of fibula
3. 腓骨颈 neck of fibula
4. 腓骨体 shaft of fibula
5. 外踝 lateral malleolus
6. 外踝窝 lateral malleolar fossa

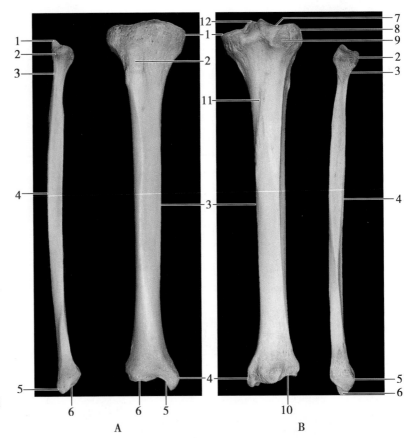

图 2-5 右侧胫骨与腓骨 Right tibia and fibula
A. 前面观 Anterior view B. 后面观 Posterior view
A 中胫骨在右，腓骨在左 Tibia is right one，fibula left one in A
B 中胫骨在左，腓骨在右 Tibia is left one，fibula right one in B

14

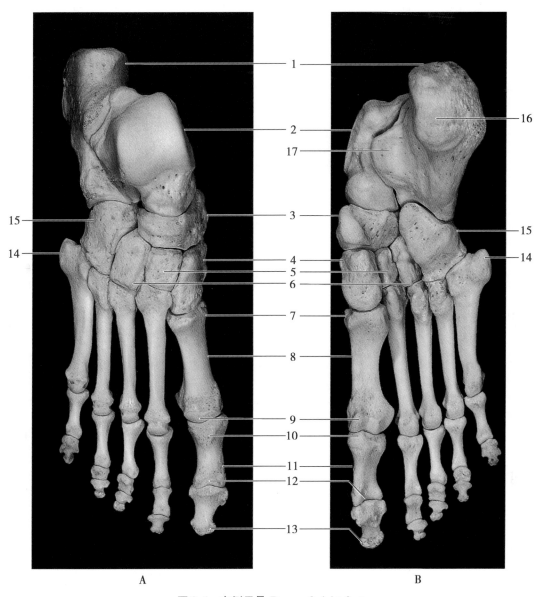

A   B

图 2-6 右侧足骨 Bones of right foot
A. 上面观 Superior view B. 下面观 Inferior view

1. 跟骨 calcaneus
2. 距骨 talus
3. 足舟骨 navicular
4. 内侧楔骨 medial cuneiform
5. 中间楔骨 intermediate cuneiform
6. 外侧楔骨 lateral cuneiform
7. 第一跖骨底 base of first metatarsal bone
8. 第一跖骨体 shaft of first metatarsal bone
9. 第一跖骨头 head of first metatarsal bone
10. 趾骨底 base of first phalanx
11. 趾骨体 shaft of first phalanx
12. 趾骨滑车 trochlea of first phalanx
13. 趾骨粗隆 tuberosity of first phalanx
14. 第五跖骨粗隆 tuberosity of fifth metatarsal bone
15. 骰骨 cuboid
16. 跟骨结节 calcaneal tuberosity
17. 载距突 sustentaculum tali

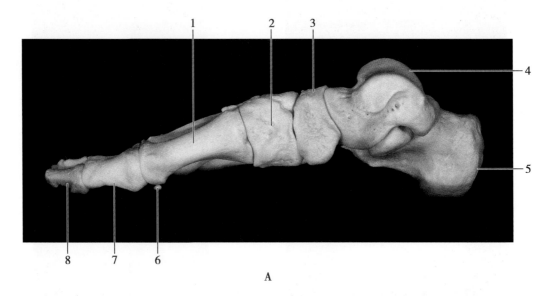

A

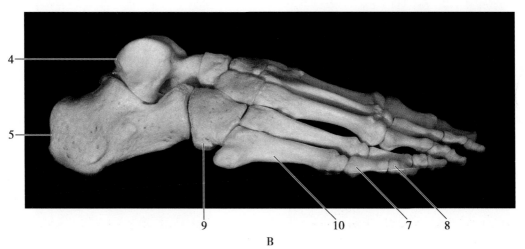

B

图 2-7 右侧足纵弓 Longitudinal arches of right foot

A. 内面观 Medial view B. 外面观 Lateral view

1. 第一跖骨 first metatarsal bone
2. 内侧楔骨 medial cuneiform
3. 足舟骨 navicular
4. 距骨 talus
5. 跟骨 calcaneus
6. 籽骨 sesamoid bone
7. 第五近节趾骨 fifth proximal phalanx
8. 第五远节趾骨 fifth distal phalanx
9. 骰骨 cuboid
10. 第五跖骨 fifth metatarsal bone

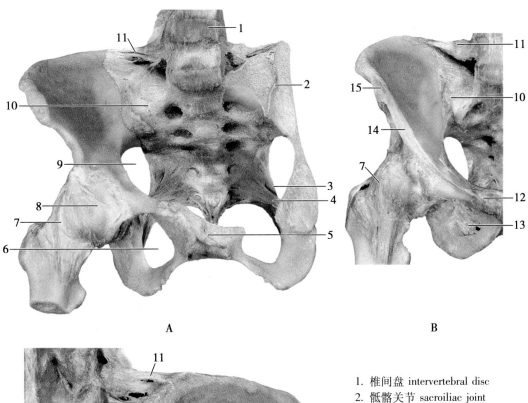

A

B

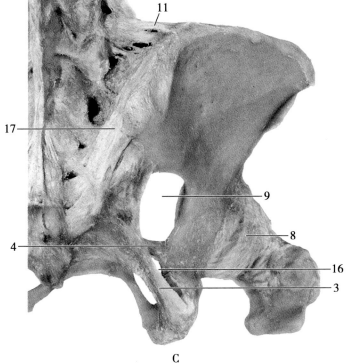

C

图 2-8 骨盆的连接 Joints of pelvis
A. 前面观 Anterior view　B. 骨盆右侧半前面观 Anterior view of
right half of pelvis　C. 后面观 Posterior view

1. 椎间盘 intervertebral disc
2. 骶髂关节 sacroiliac joint
3. 骶结节韧带 sacrotuberous ligament
4. 骶棘韧带 sacrospinous ligament
5. 耻骨联合腔 pubic symphysis cavity
6. 闭孔 obturator foramen
7. 髂股韧带 iliofemoral ligament
8. 髋关节纤维囊 fibrous capsule of hip joint
9. 坐骨大孔 greater sciatic foramen
10. 骶髂前韧带 anterior sacroiliac ligament
11. 髂腰韧带 iliolumbar ligament
12. 耻骨结节 pubic tubercle
13. 闭孔膜 obturator membrane
14. 腹股沟韧带 inguinal ligament
15. 髂前上棘 anterior superior iliac spine
16. 坐骨小孔 lesser sciatic foramen
17. 骶髂后韧带 posterior sacroiliac ligament

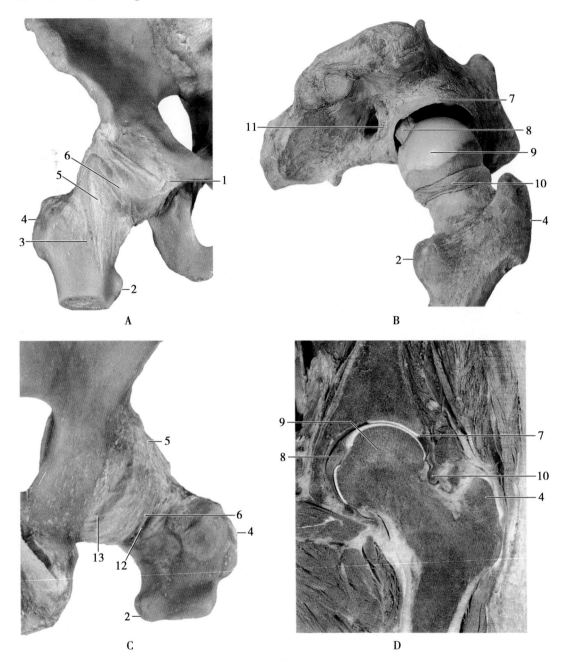

A.

B.

C.

D.

图 2-9 右髋关节 Right hip joint

A. 前面观 Anterior view B. 关节囊已切开 Dissected joint

C. 后面观 Posterior view D. 关节的冠状切面 Coronal section of joint

1. 耻骨韧带 pubofemoral ligament
2. 股骨小转子 lesser trochanter of femur
3. 转子间线 intertrochanteric line
4. 股骨大转子 greater trochanter of femur
5. 髂股韧带 iliofemoral ligament
6. 关节囊 articular capsule
7. 髋臼唇 acetabular labrum
8. 股骨头韧带 ligament of femoral head
9. 股骨头 head of femur
10. 轮匝带 zona orbicularis
11. 髋臼横韧带 transverse acetabular ligament
12. 股骨颈 neck of femur
13. 坐股韧带 ischiofemoral ligament

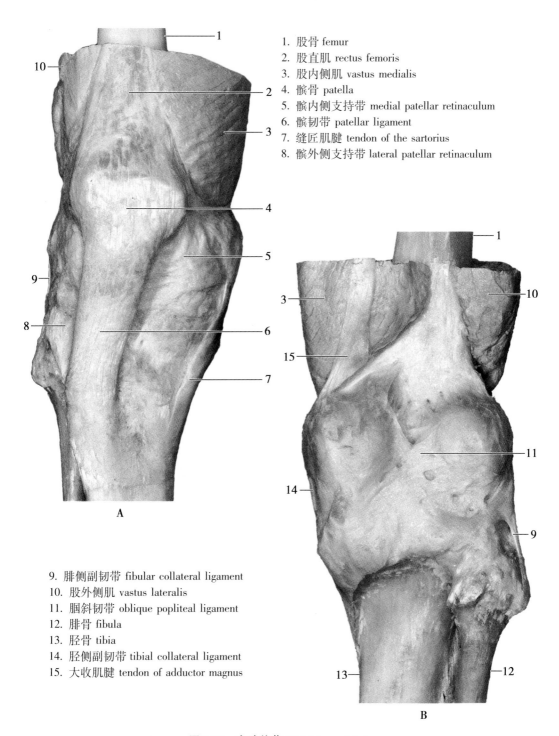

1. 股骨 femur
2. 股直肌 rectus femoris
3. 股内侧肌 vastus medialis
4. 髌骨 patella
5. 髌内侧支持带 medial patellar retinaculum
6. 髌韧带 patellar ligament
7. 缝匠肌腱 tendon of the sartorius
8. 髌外侧支持带 lateral patellar retinaculum

A

9. 腓侧副韧带 fibular collateral ligament
10. 股外侧肌 vastus lateralis
11. 腘斜韧带 oblique popliteal ligament
12. 腓骨 fibula
13. 胫骨 tibia
14. 胫侧副韧带 tibial collateral ligament
15. 大收肌腱 tendon of adductor magnus

B

图 2-10　右膝关节 Right knee joint
A. 前面观 Anterior view　B. 后面观 Posterior view

19

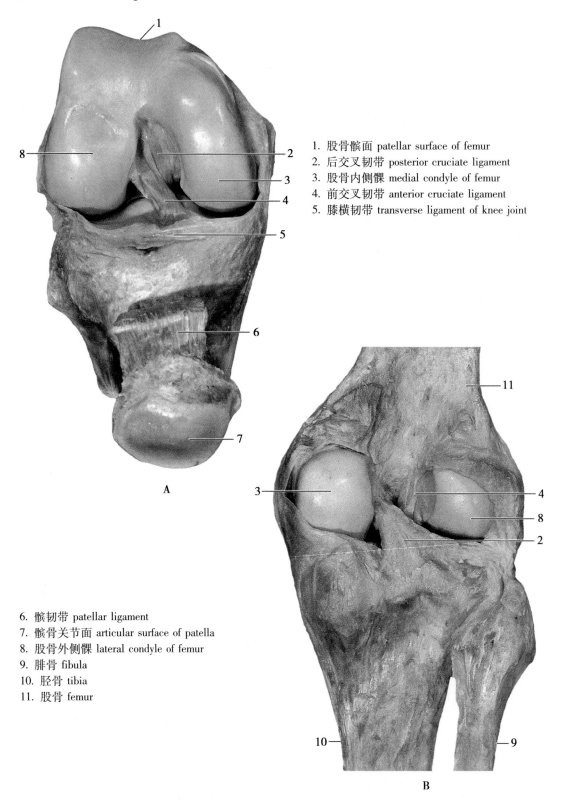

1. 股骨髌面 patellar surface of femur
2. 后交叉韧带 posterior cruciate ligament
3. 股骨内侧髁 medial condyle of femur
4. 前交叉韧带 anterior cruciate ligament
5. 膝横韧带 transverse ligament of knee joint

6. 髌韧带 patellar ligament
7. 髌骨关节面 articular surface of patella
8. 股骨外侧髁 lateral condyle of femur
9. 腓骨 fibula
10. 胫骨 tibia
11. 股骨 femur

图 2-11　剖开的右膝关节 Dissected right knee joint
A. 前面观 Anterior view　B. 后面观 Posterior view

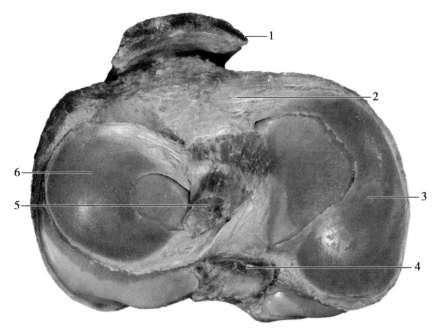

图 2-12　右侧膝关节半月板(上面观) Meniscuses of right knee joint(superior view)

1. 髌韧带 patellar ligament
2. 膝横韧带 transverse ligament of knee joint
3. 内侧半月板 medial meniscus
4. 后交叉韧带 posterior cruciate ligament
5. 前交叉韧带 anterior cruciate ligament
6. 外侧半月板 lateral meniscus

图 2-13　右侧膝关节矢状切面
Sagittal section through right knee joint

1. 股骨 femur
2. 髌上囊 suprapatellar bursa
3. 股四头肌腱 tendon of quadriceps femoris
4. 髌骨 patella
5. 翼状襞 alar folds
6. 髌韧带 patellar ligament
7. 胫骨 tibia

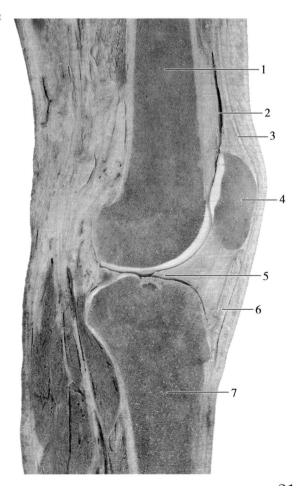

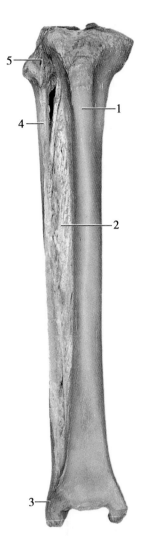

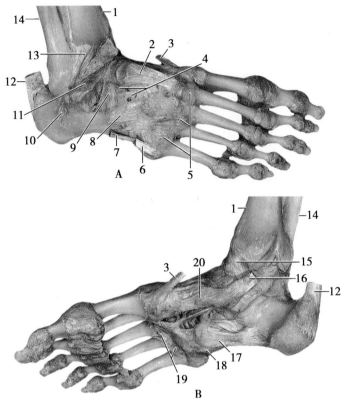

图 2-14　右侧小腿骨连接
（前面观）
Joints of right leg
（anterior view）

1. 胫骨 tibia
2. 小腿骨间膜 crural interosseous membrane
3. 胫腓前韧带 anterior tibiofibular ligament
4. 腓骨 fibula
5. 胫腓关节 tibiofibular joint

图 2-15　右侧踝关节周围的韧带
Ligaments around right ankle joint

A. 上面观 Superior view　B. 下面观 Inferior view

1. 胫骨 tibia
2. 楔舟背侧韧带 dorsal cuneonavicular ligament
3. 胫骨前肌腱 tendon of the tibialis anterior
4. 分歧韧带 bifurcated ligament
5. 跗跖背侧韧带 dorsal tarsometatarsal ligament
6. 腓骨短肌腱 tendon of peroneus brevis
7. 腓骨长肌腱 tendon of peroneus longus
8. 跟骰背侧韧带 dorsal calcaneocuboid ligament
9. 距跟骨间韧带 interosseous talocalcaneal ligament
10. 跟腓韧带 calcaneofibular ligament
11. 距腓前韧带 anterior talofibular ligament
12. 跟腱 tendo calcaneus
13. 胫腓前韧带 anterior tibiofibular ligament
14. 腓骨 fibula
15. 内侧（三角）韧带 medial（deltoid）ligament
16. 胫骨后肌腱 tendon of tibialis posterior
17. 足底长韧带 long plantar ligament
18. 腓骨长肌腱 tendon of peroneus longus
19. 跖骨足底韧带 plantar metatarsal ligament
20. 跗跖足底韧带 plantar tarsometatarsal ligament

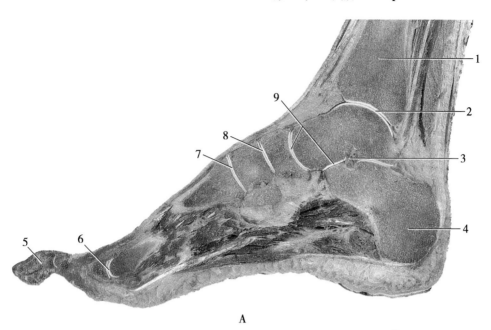

A

1. 胫骨 tibia
2. 距小腿关节（踝关节） talocrural（ankle）joint
3. 距跟骨间韧带 interosseous talocalcaneal ligament
4. 跟骨 calcaneus
5. 趾骨间关节 interphalangeal joint
6. 跖趾关节 metatarsophalangeal joint
7. 跗跖关节 tarsometatarsal joint
8. 楔舟关节 cuneonavicular joint
9. 距跟舟关节 talocalcaneonavicular joint
10. 跖骨间关节 intermetatarsal joint
11. 跟骰关节 calcaneocuboid joint
12. 腓骨 fibula

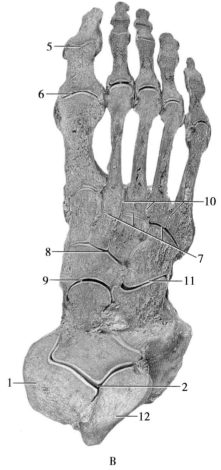

B

图 2-16　右侧足骨关节 Joints of right foot
A. 矢状切面 Sagittal section through joints　B. 横切面 Transverse section through joints

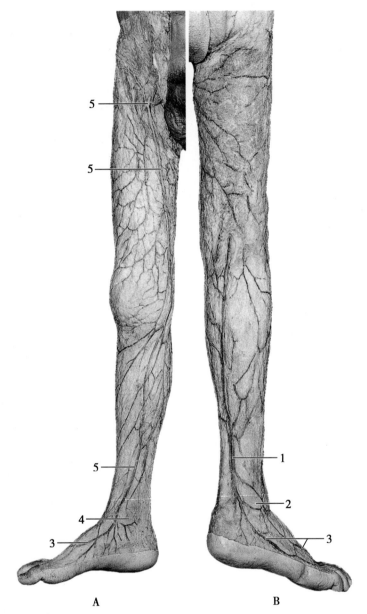

图 2-17　右下肢浅静脉 Superficial veins of the right lower limb

A. 内侧面观 Medial view　　B. 外侧面观 Lateral view

1. 小隐静脉 small saphenous vein　　4. 胫骨内踝 medial malleolus of tibia
2. 腓骨外踝 lateral malleolus of fibula　　5. 大隐静脉 great saphenous vein
3. 足背静脉弓 dorsal venous arch of foot

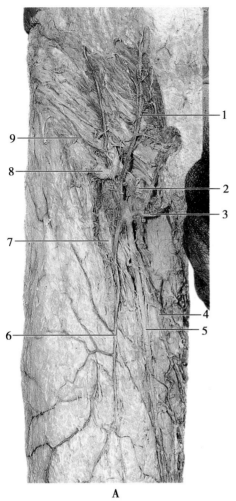

A

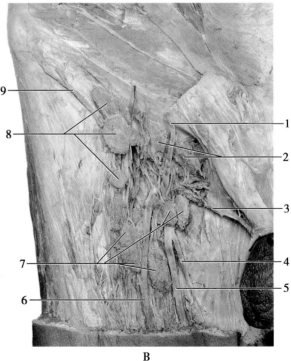

1. 腹壁浅静脉 superficial epigastric vein
2. 腹股沟上内侧浅淋巴结 superomedial superficial inguinal lymph nodes
3. 阴部外静脉 external pudendal vein
4. 股内侧浅静脉 medial superficial femoral vein
5. 大隐静脉 great saphenous vein
6. 股外侧浅静脉 lateral superficial femoral vein
7. 腹股沟下浅淋巴结 inferior superficial inguinal lymph nodes
8. 腹股沟上外侧浅淋巴结 superolateral superficial inguinal lymph nodes
9. 旋髂浅静脉 superficial circumflex iliac vein

B

图 2-18　右股前内侧区的浅层结构 Superficial structures of anteromedial region of the right thigh
A. 浅静脉 Superficial veins　B. 浅淋巴结 Superficial lymph nodes

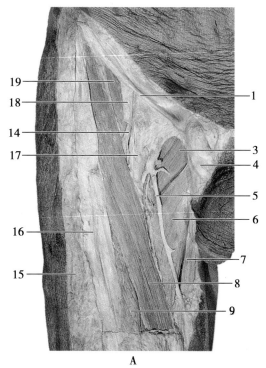

A

1. 腹股沟韧带 inguinal ligament
2. 股静脉 femoral vein
3. 耻骨肌 pectineus
4. 精索 spermatic cord
5. 大隐静脉 great saphenous vein
6. 长收肌 adductor longus
7. 股薄肌 gracilis
8. 缝匠肌 sartorius
9. 股直肌 rectus femoris
10. 股内侧肌 vastus medialis

11. 股外侧肌 vastus lateralis
12. 阔筋膜张肌 tensor fasciae latae
13. 股动脉 femoral artery
14. 股神经 femoral nerve
15. 浅筋膜 superficial fascia
16. 阔筋膜 fascia lata
17. 股鞘 femoral sheath
18. 髂筋膜 iliac fascia
19. 髂腰肌 iliopsoas

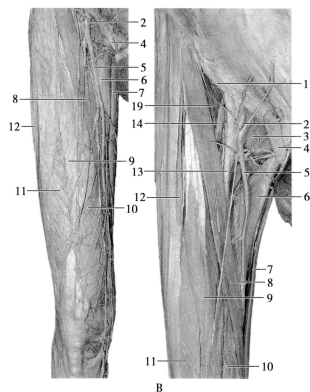

B

图 2-19 　右股前内侧区的深层结构（Ⅰ）**Deep structures in anteromedial region of right thigh**（Ⅰ）
A. 股鞘 Femoral sheath　B. 股三角的肌、神经、血管 Muscles, nerves and blood vessels in femoral triangle

26

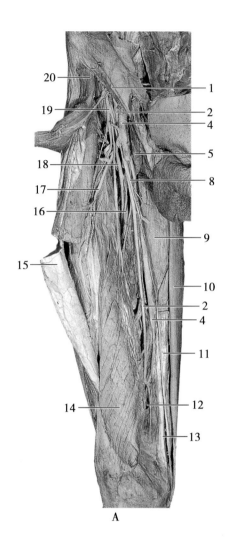

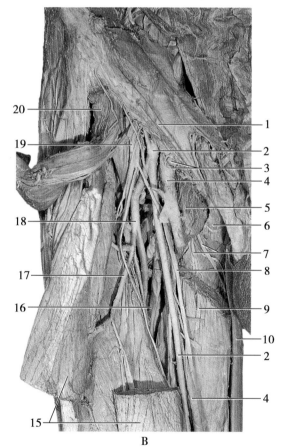

1. 腹股沟韧带 inguinal ligament
2. 股动脉 femoral artery
3. 股管及腹股沟深淋巴结 femoral canal and deep inguinal lymph nodes
4. 股静脉 femoral vein
5. 耻骨肌 pectineus
6. 短收肌 adductor brevis
7. 闭孔神经前支 anterior branch of obturator nerve
8. 隐神经 saphenous nerve
9. 长收肌 adductor longus
10. 股薄肌 gracilis
11. 大收肌 adductor magnus
12. 收肌腱裂孔 adductor hiatus

13. 大收肌腱 tendon of adductor magnus
14. 股内侧肌 vastus medialis
15. 股直肌 rectus femoris
16. 股深静脉 deep femoral vein
17. 旋股外侧动脉 lateral circumflex femoral artery
18. 股深动脉 deep femoral artery
19. 股神经 femoral nerve
20. 缝匠肌 sartorius

图 2-20　右股前内侧区的深层结构（Ⅱ）
Deep structures in anteromedial region of right thigh（Ⅱ）
A. 收肌管 Adductor canal　B. 股深动脉及其分支 Deep femoral artery and its branches

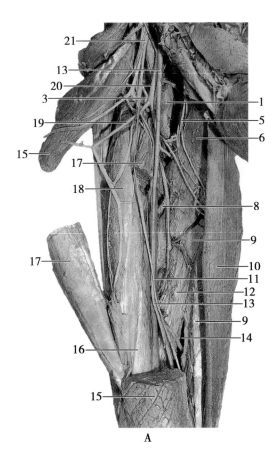

1. 耻骨肌 pectineus
2. 股静脉 femoral vein
3. 旋股内侧动脉 medial circumflex femoral artery
4. 闭孔外肌 obturator externus
5. 闭孔神经 obturator nerve
6. 短收肌 adductor brevis
7. 股深静脉 deep femoral vein
8. 穿动脉 perforating artery
9. 大收肌 adductor magnus
10. 股薄肌 gracilis
11. 隐神经 saphenous nerve

A

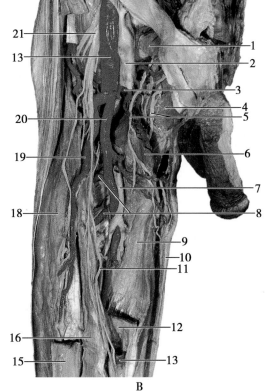

B

12. 长收肌 adductor longus
13. 股动脉 femoral artery
14. 收肌腱裂孔 adductor hiatus
15. 股直肌 rectus femoris
16. 股内侧肌 vastus medialis
17. 股中间肌 vastus intermedius
18. 股外侧肌 vastus lateralis
19. 旋股外侧动脉 lateral circumflex femoral artery
20. 股深动脉 deep femoral artery
21. 股神经 femoral nerve

图 2-21　右股前内侧区的深层结构(Ⅲ)
Deep structures in anteromedial region of right thigh(Ⅲ)
A. 股动脉及其分支 Femoral artery and its branches
B. 股深动脉及其穿支 Deep femoral artery and its perforating branches

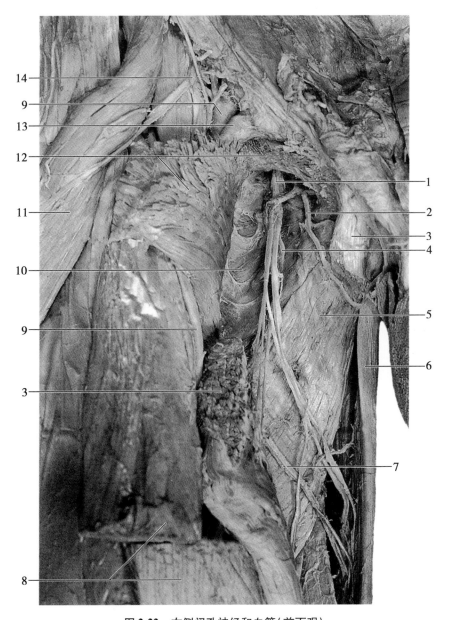

图 2-22 右侧闭孔神经和血管（前面观）
Right Obturator nerves and vessels（anterior view）

1. 闭孔神经 obturator nerve
2. 闭孔动脉前支 anterior branch of obturator artery
3. 长收肌 adductor longus
4. 闭孔动脉后支 posterior branch of obturator artery
5. 短收肌 adductor brevis
6. 股薄肌 gracilis
7. 旋股内侧动脉深支 deep branch of medial circumflex femoral artery

8. 股直肌 rectus femoris
9. 股动脉 femoral artery
10. 闭孔外肌 obturator externus
11. 缝匠肌 sartorius
12. 耻骨肌 pectineus
13. 股静脉 femoral vein
14. 股神经 femoral nerve

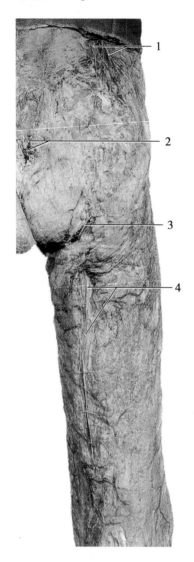

图 2-24　右侧臀区和股后区的肌
Muscles of right gluteal region and
posterior region of thigh

图 2-23　右侧臀区和股后区的皮神经
Cutaneous nerves of right gluteal region and
posterior region of thigh

1. 臀上皮神经 superior clunial nerve
2. 臀内侧皮神经 medial clunial nerve
3. 臀下皮神经 inferior clunial nerve
4. 股后皮神经 posterior femoral cutaneous nerve

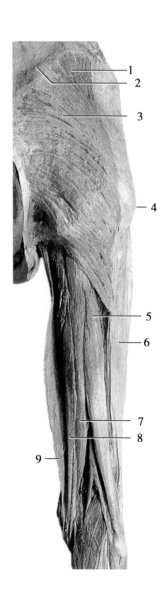

图 2-24　右侧臀区和股后区的肌
Muscles of right gluteal region and
posterior region of thigh

1. 臀中肌 gluteus medius
2. 髂后上棘 posterior superior iliac spine
3. 臀大肌 gluteus maximus
4. 股骨大转子 greater trochanter of femur
5. 股二头肌 biceps femoris
6. 髂胫束 iliotibial tract
7. 半膜肌 semimembranosus
8. 半腱肌 semitendinosus
9. 股薄肌 gracilis

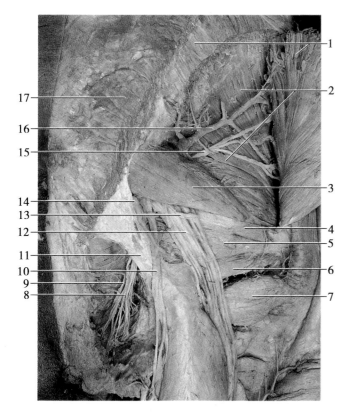

图 2-25　右侧臀区的肌、神经和血管（Ⅰ）
Muscles, nerves and blood vessels of right gluteal region（Ⅰ）

1. 臀中肌 gluteus medius
2. 臀小肌 gluteus minimus
3. 梨状肌 piriformis
4. 上孖肌 gemellus superior
5. 闭孔内肌腱 tendon of obturator internus
6. 下孖肌 gemellus inferior
7. 股方肌 quadratus femoris
8. 阴部神经 pudendal nerve
9. 阴部内动脉 internal pudendal artery

图 2-26　右侧臀区的肌、神经和血管（Ⅱ）
Muscles, nerves and blood vessels of right gluteal region（Ⅱ）

10. 股后皮神经 posterior femoral cutaneous nerve
11. 骶结节韧带 sacrotuberous ligament
12. 坐骨神经 sciatic nerve
13. 臀下神经 inferior gluteal nerve
14. 臀下动脉 inferior gluteal artery
15. 臀上神经 superior gluteal nerve
16. 臀上动脉 superior gluteal artery
17. 臀大肌 gluteus maximus

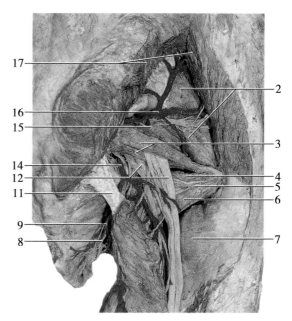

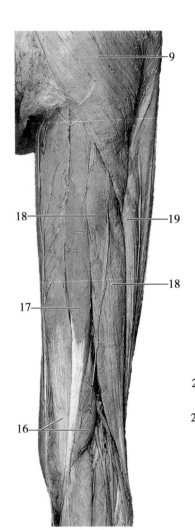

图 2-27 右股后区的肌
Muscles of posterior region
of right thigh

1. 臀中肌 gluteus medius
2. 梨状肌 piriformis
3. 上孖肌 gemellus superior
4. 闭孔内肌腱 tendon of obturator internus
5. 下孖肌 gemellus inferior
6. 股方肌 quadratus femoris
7. 旋股内侧动脉 medial circumflex femoral artery
8. 臀下动脉 inferior gluteal artery
9. 臀大肌 gluteus maximus
10. 大收肌 adductor magnus
11. 第一穿动脉 first perforating artery
12. 第二穿动脉 second perforating artery

13. 第三穿动脉 third perforating artery
14. 坐骨神经 sciatic nerve
15. 股二头肌短头 short head of biceps femoris
16. 半膜肌 semimembranosus
17. 半腱肌 semitendinosus
18. 股二头肌长头 long head of biceps femoris
19. 阔筋膜张肌 tensor fasciae latae
20. 股后皮神经 posterior femoral cutaneous nerve
21. 骶结韧带 sacrotuberous ligament

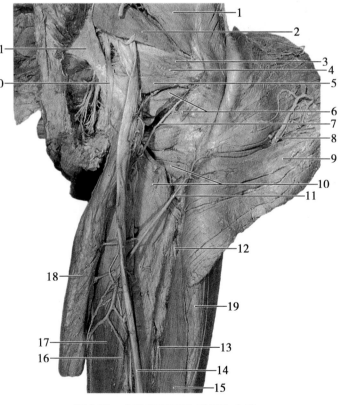

图 2-28 右股后区的肌、神经和血管
Muscles, nerves and blood vessels of posterior
region of right thigh

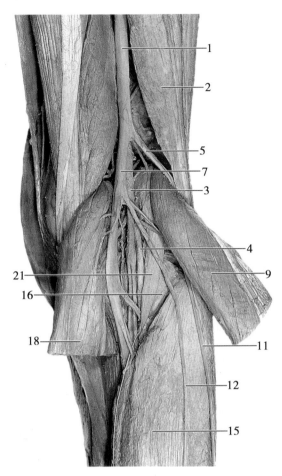

1. 坐骨神经 sciatic nerve
2. 股二头肌 biceps femoris
3. 腘静脉 popliteal vein
4. 腘动脉 popliteal artery
5. 腓总神经 common peroneal nerve
6. 膝上外侧动脉 lateral superior genicular artery
7. 胫神经 tibial nerve
8. 小隐静脉 small saphenous vein
9. 腓肠肌外侧头 lateral head of gastrocnemius
10. 膝下外侧动脉 lateral inferior genicular artery
11. 腓肠外侧皮神经 lateral sural cutaneous nerve

图 2-29 右腘窝的神经和血管
Nerves and blood vessels in right popliteal fossa

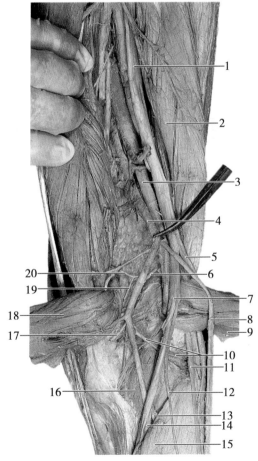

图 2-30 右腘动脉及其分支
Branches of right popliteal artery

12. 腓肠内侧皮神经 medial sural cutaneous nerve
13. 胫前动脉 anterior tibial artery
14. 胫后动脉 posterior tibial artery
15. 比目鱼肌 soleus
16. 腘肌 popliteus
17. 膝下内侧动脉 medial inferior genicular artery
18. 腓肠肌内侧头 medial head of gastrocnemius
19. 膝中动脉 middle genicular artery
20. 膝上内侧动脉 medial superior genicular artery
21. 跖肌 plantaris

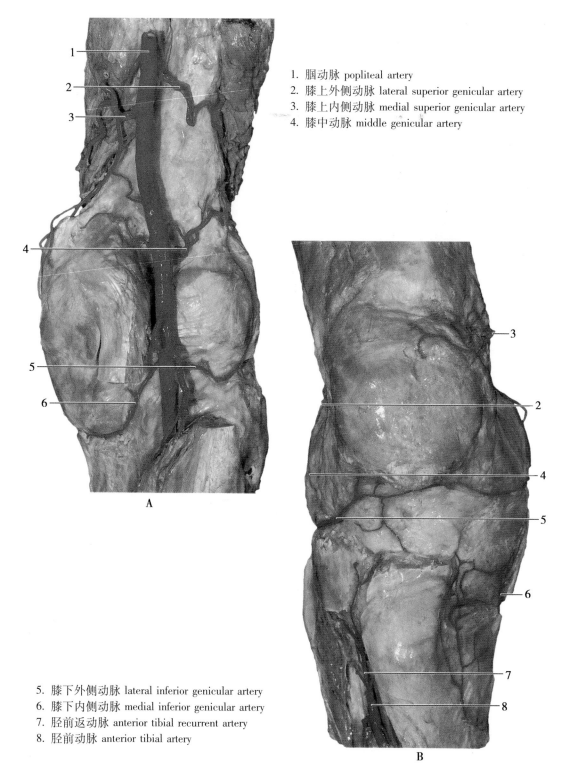

1. 腘动脉 popliteal artery
2. 膝上外侧动脉 lateral superior genicular artery
3. 膝上内侧动脉 medial superior genicular artery
4. 膝中动脉 middle genicular artery

5. 膝下外侧动脉 lateral inferior genicular artery
6. 膝下内侧动脉 medial inferior genicular artery
7. 胫前返动脉 anterior tibial recurrent artery
8. 胫前动脉 anterior tibial artery

A

B

图 2-31　右膝关节动脉网 Right genicular arterial anastmosis
A. 前面观 Anterior view　B. 后面观 Posterior view

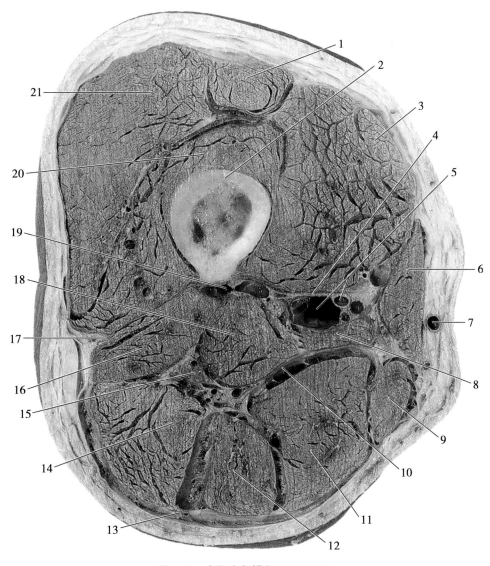

图 2-32　右股中部横断面（下面观）
Transverse section through middle of right thigh (inferior view)

1. 股直肌 rectus femoris
2. 股骨 femur
3. 股内侧肌 vastus medialis
4. 股内侧肌间隔 medial femoral intermuscular septum
5. 股动脉、股静脉 femoral artery and vein
6. 缝匠肌 sartorius
7. 大隐静脉 great saphenous vein
8. 长收肌 adductor longus
9. 股薄肌 gracilis
10. 股后肌间隔 posterior femoral intermuscular septum
11. 半膜肌 semimembranosus
12. 半腱肌 semitendinosus
13. 股后皮神经 posterior femoral cutaneous nerve
14. 股二头肌长头 long head of biceps femoris
15. 坐骨神经 sciatic nerve
16. 股二头肌短头 short head of biceps femoris
17. 股外侧肌间隔 lateral femoral intermuscular septum
18. 大收肌 adductor magnus
19. 股深动脉及穿动脉 deep femoral artery and perforating artery
20. 股中间肌 vastus intermedius
21. 股外侧肌 vastus lateralis

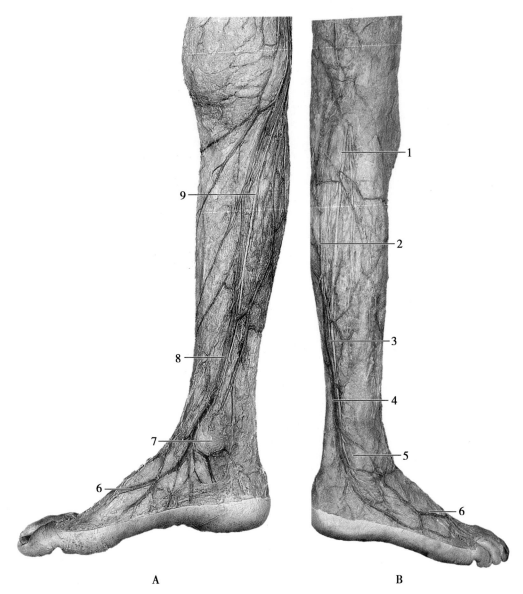

A   B

图 2-33 右小腿浅静脉 Superficial veins of right leg
A. 内侧观 Medial view B. 外侧观 Lateral view

1. 腓肠外侧皮神经 lateral sural cutaneous nerve
2. 腓肠内侧皮神经 medial sural cutaneous nerve
3. 腓肠神经 sural nerve
4. 小隐静脉 small saphenous vein
5. 腓骨外踝 lateral malleolus of fibula
6. 足背静脉弓 dorsal venous arch of foot
7. 胫骨内踝 medial malleolus of tibia
8. 大隐静脉 great saphenous vein
9. 隐神经 saphenous nerve

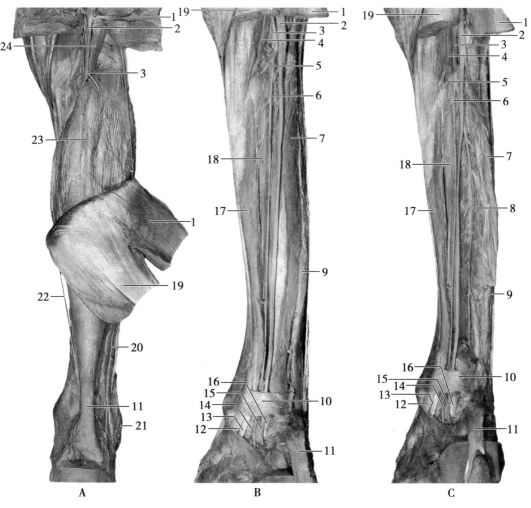

A　　　　　　　　B　　　　　　　　C

图 2-34　右小腿后区结构 Structures in posterior compartment of right leg

A. 浅层 Superficial layer　B. 中层 Middle layer　C. 深层 Deep layer

1. 腓肠肌外侧头 lateral head of gastrocnemius
2. 胫神经 tibial nerve
3. 腘动脉 popliteal artery
4. 腘静脉 popliteal vein
5. 胫前动脉 anterior tibial artery
6. 胫后动脉 posterior tibial artery
7. 蹈长屈肌 flexor hallucis longus
8. 腓动脉 peroneal artery
9. 腓骨长肌 peroneus longus
10. 屈肌支持带 flexor retinaculum
11. 跟腱 tendo calcaneus
12. 胫骨后肌腱 tendon of tibialis posterior

13. 趾长屈肌腱 tendon of flexor digitorum longus
14. 胫后动脉 posterior tibial artery
15. 胫神经 tibial nerve
16. 蹈长屈肌腱 tendon of flexor hallucis longus
17. 趾长屈肌 flexor digitorum longus
18. 胫骨后肌 tibialis posterior
19. 腓肠肌内侧头 medial head of gastrocnemius
20. 大隐静脉 great saphenous vein
21. 腓骨外踝 lateral malleolus of fibula
22. 跖肌腱 tendon of plantaris
23. 比目鱼肌 soleus
24. 跖肌 plantaris

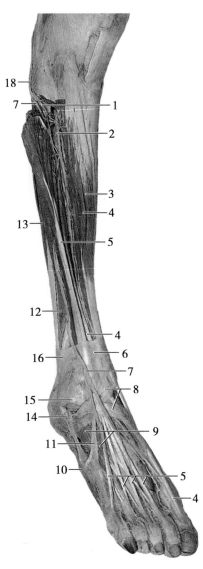

1. 腓深神经 deep peroneal nerve
2. 胫前动脉 anterior tibial artery
3. 胫骨前肌 tibialis anterior
4. 踇长伸肌 extensor hallucis longus
5. 趾长伸肌 extensor digitorum longus
6. 伸肌上支持带 superior extensor retinaculum
7. 腓浅神经 superficial peroneal nerve
8. 伸肌下支持带 inferior extensor retinaculum
9. 趾短伸肌 extensor digitorum brevis
10. 第五跖骨粗隆 tuberosity of fifth metatarsal bone
11. 第三腓骨肌腱 tendon of peroneus tertius

图 2-35 右小腿前外侧区和足背
Anterolateral compartment of right leg
and dorsum of foot

12. 腓骨短肌腱 tendon of peroneus brevis
13. 腓骨长肌腱 tendon of peroneus longus
14. 腓骨肌下支持带 inferior peroneal retinaculum
15. 腓骨外踝 lateral malleolus of fibula
16. 腓骨肌上支持带 superior peroneal retinaculum
17. 跟腱 tendo calcaneus
18. 腓总神经 common peroneal nerve

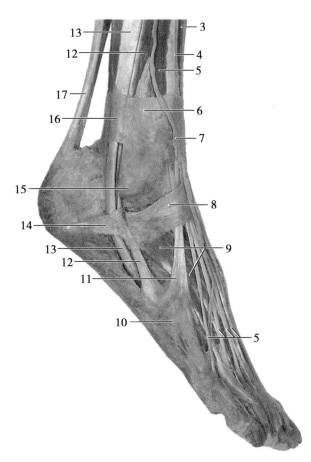

图 2-36 右小腿伸肌支持带和腓骨肌支持带
Right extensor retinaculum and
peroneal retinaculum

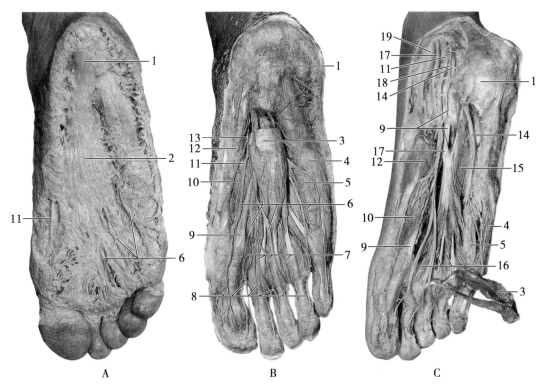

图 2-37　右足底结构（Ⅰ）Structures of sole of right foot（Ⅰ）

A. 足底腱膜 Plantar aponeurosis　B. 浅层肌、神经和血管 Superficial muscles, nerves and blood vessels
C. 足底中层的肌、血管和神经 Middle muscles, nerves and blood vessels

1. 跟骨 calcaneus
2. 足底腱膜 plantar aponeurosis
3. 趾短屈肌 flexor digitorum brevis
4. 小趾展肌 abductor digiti minimi
5. 小趾短屈肌 flexor digiti minimi brevis
6. 趾足底总神经 common plantar digital nerve
7. 趾足底总动脉 common plantar digital artery
8. 趾足底固有动脉 proper plantar digital artery
9. 姆长屈肌腱 tendon of flexor hallucis longus
10. 姆短屈肌 flexor hallucis brevis

11. 足底内侧神经 medial plantar nerve
12. 姆展肌 abductor hallucis
13. 足底内侧动脉 medial plantar artery
14. 足底外侧神经 lateral plantar nerve
15. 足底方肌 quadratus plantae
16. 蚓状肌 lumbricals
17. 趾长屈肌腱 tendon of flexor digitorum longus
18. 胫后动脉 posterior tibial artery
19. 胫骨后肌腱 tendon of tibialis posterior

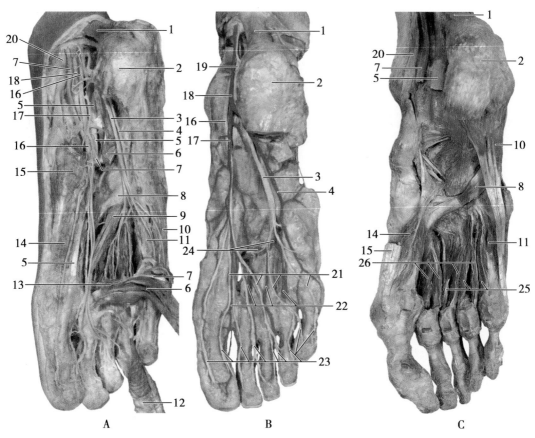

图 2-38　右足底结构(Ⅱ) Structures of sole of right foot(Ⅱ)

A、B. 神经和血管 Nerves and blood vessels　C. 肌 Muscles

1. 跟腱 tendo calcaneus
2. 跟骨 calcaneus
3. 足底外侧神经 lateral plantar nerve
4. 足底外侧动脉 lateral plantar artery
5. 踇长屈肌腱 tendon of flexor hallucis longus
6. 足底方肌 quadratus plantae
7. 趾长屈肌腱 tendon of flexor digitorum longus
8. 腓骨长肌腱 tendon of peroneus longus
9. 踇收肌(斜头) adductor hallucis(oblique head)
10. 小趾展肌 abductor digiti minimi
11. 小趾短屈肌 flexor digiti minimi brevis
12. 趾短屈肌 flexor digitorum brevis
13. 踇收肌(横头) adductor hallucis(transverse head)
14. 踇短屈肌 flexor hallucis brevis
15. 踇展肌 abductor hallucis
16. 足底内侧神经 medial plantar nerve
17. 足底内侧动脉 medial plantar artery
18. 胫后动脉 posterior tibial artery
19. 胫神经 tibial nerve
20. 胫骨后肌腱 tendon of tibialis posterior
21. 趾足底总神经 common plantar digital nerve
22. 趾足底总动脉 common plantar digital artery
23. 趾足底固有神经、动脉 proper plantar digital nerve and artery
24. 足底深弓 deep plantar arch
25. 骨间足底肌 plantar interossei
26. 骨间背侧肌 dorsal interossei

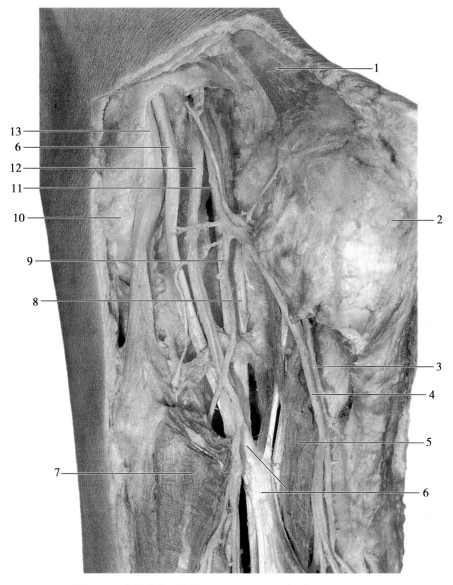

图 2-39　右踝管(下面观) Right tarsal tunnel(inferior view)

1. 跟腱 tendo calcaneus
2. 跟骨 calcaneus
3. 足底外侧动脉 lateral plantar artery
4. 足底外侧神经 lateral plantar nerve
5. 足底方肌 quadratus platae
6. 趾长屈肌腱 tendon of flexor digitorum longus
7. 蹬展肌 abductor hallucis
8. 蹬长屈肌腱 tendon of flexor hallucis longus
9. 足底内侧动脉 medial plantar artery
10. 胫骨内踝 medial malleolus of tibia
11. 胫后动脉 posterior tibial artery
12. 足底内侧神经 medial plantar nerve
13. 胫骨后肌腱 tendon of tibialis posterior

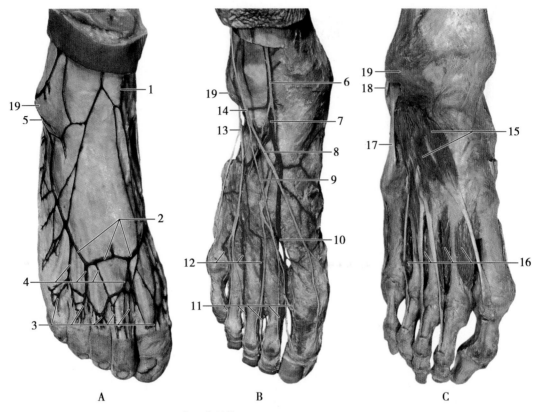

图 2-40　右足背结构 Structures of dorsum of right foot

A. 浅静脉 Superficial veins　B. 神经和动脉 Nerves and arteries　C. 肌 Muscles

1. 大隐静脉 great saphenous vein
2. 足背静脉弓 dorsal venous arch of foot
3. 趾背静脉 dorsal digital vein of foot
4. 跖背静脉 dorsal metatarsal vein
5. 小隐静脉 small saphenous vein
6. 腓深神经 deep peroneal nerve
7. 足背动脉 dorsal artery of foot
8. 足背内侧皮神经 medial dorsal cutaneous nerve of foot
9. 足背中间皮神经 intermediate dorsal cutaneous nerve of foot
10. 第一跖背动脉 first dorsal metatarsal artery

11. 趾背神经和动脉 dorsal digital nerve and artery of foot
12. 跖背动脉 dorsal metatarsal artery
13. 足背外侧皮神经 lateral dorsal cutaneous nerve of foot
14. 腓浅神经 superficial peroneal nerve
15. 趾短伸肌 extensor digitorum brevis
16. 骨间背侧肌 dorsal interossei
17. 腓骨短肌腱 tendon of peroneus brevis
18. 腓骨长肌腱 tendon of peroneus longus
19. 腓骨外踝 lateral malleolus of fibula

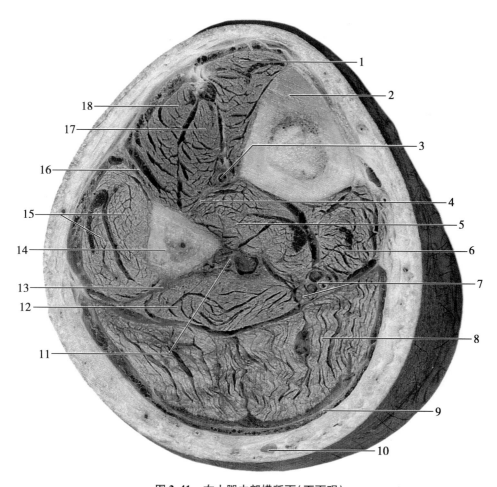

图 2-41　右小腿中部横断面(下面观)
Transverse section through middle of right leg(inferior view)

1. 胫骨前肌 tibialis anterior
2. 胫骨 tibia
3. 胫前动脉 anterior tibial artery
4. 小腿骨间膜 crural interosseous membrane
5. 胫骨后肌 tibialis posterior
6. 趾长屈肌 flexor digitorum longus
7. 胫神经及胫后动脉 tibial nerve and posterior tibial artery
8. 比目鱼肌 soleus
9. 腓肠肌腱膜 aponeurosis of gastrocnemius
10. 小隐静脉 small saphenous vein
11. 腓动脉、静脉 peroneal artery and vein
12. 姆长屈肌 flexor hallucis longus
13. 小腿后肌间隔 posterior crural intermuscular septum
14. 腓骨 fibula
15. 腓骨长肌和短肌 peroneus longus and brevis
16. 小腿前肌间隔 anterior crural intermuscular septum
17. 姆长伸肌 extensor hallucis longus
18. 趾长伸肌 extensor digitorum longus

第 3 章　上肢

Chapter 3　Upper Limb

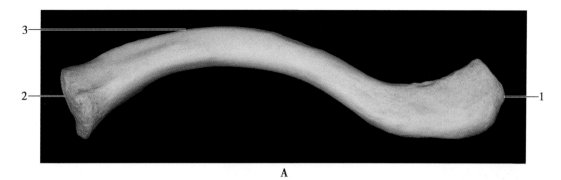

A

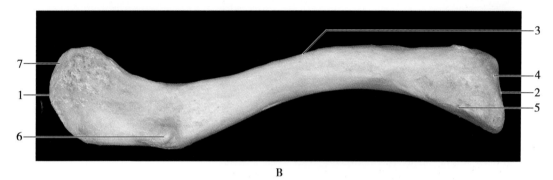

B

图 3-1　右锁骨 Right clavicle

A. 上面观 Superior view　B. 下面观 Inferior view

1. 肩峰端 acromial end
2. 胸骨端 sternal end
3. 锁骨体 shaft of clavicle
4. 胸骨关节面 sternal articular facet
5. 肋锁韧带压迹 impression for costoclavicular ligament
6. 锥状结节 conoid tubercle
7. 肩峰关节面 acromial articular facet

图 3-2　右肩胛骨外侧角
Lateral angle of right scapula

1. 喙突 coracoid process
2. 盂上结节 supraglenoid tubercle
3. 关节盂 glenoid cavity
4. 盂下结节 infraglenoid tubercle
5. 肩峰角 acromial angle
6. 肩峰 acromion

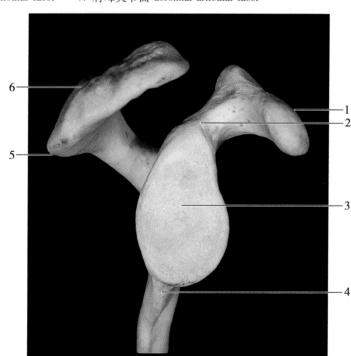

45

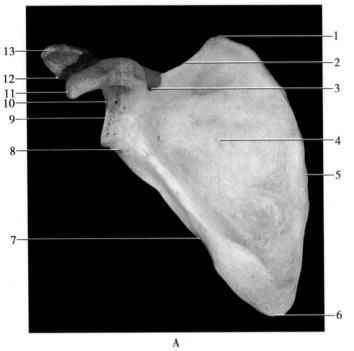

A

图 3-3　右肩胛骨 **Right scapula**
    A. 前面观 Anterior view
    B. 后面观 Posterior view
1. 上角 superior angle
2. 上缘 superior border
3. 肩胛上切迹 suprascapular notch
4. 肩胛下窝 subscapular fossa
5. 内侧缘 medial border
6. 下角 inferior angle

7. 外侧缘 lateral border
8. 盂下结节 infraglenoid tubercle
9. 关节盂 glenoid cavity
10. 盂上结节 supraglenoid tubercle
11. 喙突 coracoid process
12. 肩峰角 acromial angle
13. 肩峰 acromion
14. 肩胛颈 neck of scapula
15. 冈下窝 infraspinous fossa
16. 肩胛冈 spine of scapula
17. 冈上窝 supraspinous fossa

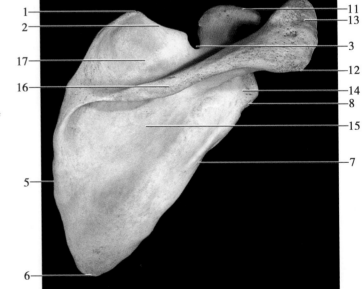

B

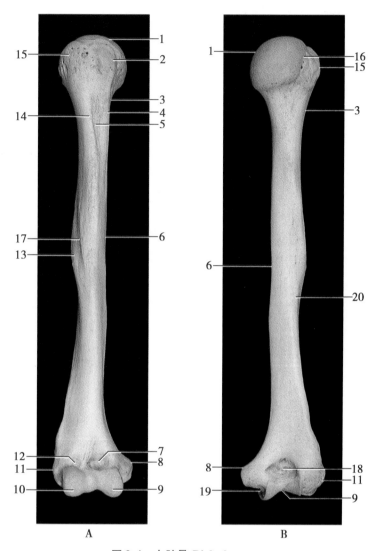

A

B

图 3-4　右肱骨 Right humerus

A. 前面观 Anterior view　B. 后面观 Posterior view

1. 肱骨头 head of humerus
2. 小结节 lesser tubercle
3. 外科颈 surgical neck
4. 小结节嵴 crest of lesser tubercle
5. 结节间沟 intertubercular sulcus
6. 肱骨体 shaft of humerus
7. 冠突窝 coronoid fossa
8. 内上髁 medial epicondyle
9. 肱骨滑车 trochlea of humerus
10. 肱骨小头 capitulum of humerus
11. 外上髁 lateral epicondyle
12. 桡窝 radial fossa
13. 三角肌粗隆 deltoid tuberosity
14. 大结节嵴 crest of greater tubercle
15. 大结节 greater tubercle
16. 解剖颈 anatomical neck
17. 桡神经沟 radial groove
18. 鹰嘴窝 olecranon fossa
19. 尺神经沟 sulcus for ulnar nerve
20. 外上髁上嵴 lateral supraepicondylar ridge

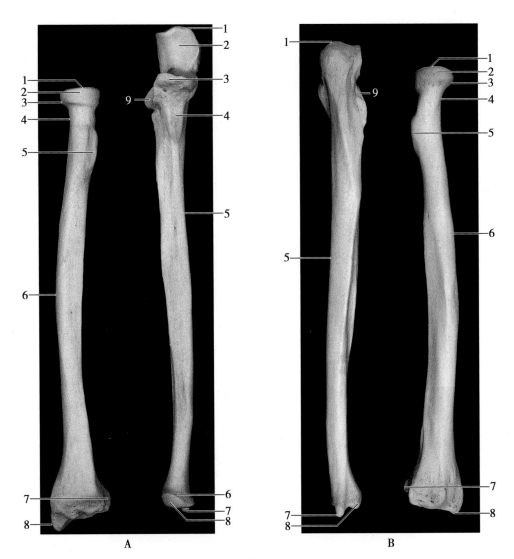

图 3-5　右桡骨和尺骨 Right radius and ulna

A. 前面观 Anterior view　B. 后面观 Posterior view

A 中桡骨在左, 尺骨在右; B 中桡骨在右, 尺骨在左 Radius is left one, ulna right one in A;

radius is right one, ulna left one in B

桡骨 Radius

1. 关节凹 articular fovea
2. 环状关节面 articular circumference
3. 桡骨头 head of radius
4. 桡骨颈 neck or radius
5. 桡骨粗隆 radial tuberosity
6. 桡骨体 shaft of radius
7. 尺切迹 ulnar notch
8. 桡骨茎突 styloid process of radius

尺骨 Ulna

1. 鹰嘴 olecranon
2. 滑车切迹 trochlear notch
3. 冠突 coronoid process
4. 尺骨粗隆 ulnar tuberosity
5. 尺骨体 shaft of ulna
6. 尺骨头 head of ulna
7. 尺骨茎突 styloid process of ulna
8. 环状关节面 articular circumference
9. 桡切迹 radial notch

48

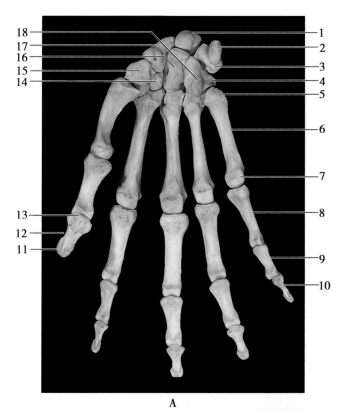

A

1. 月骨 lunate
2. 豌豆骨 pisiform
3. 三角骨 triquetrum
4. 钩骨 hamate
5. 第五掌骨底 base of fifth metacarpal
6. 第五掌骨体 shaft of fifth metacarpal
7. 第五掌骨头 head of fifth metacarpal
8. 第五近节指骨 fifth proximal phalanx
9. 第五中节指骨 fifth middle phalanx
10. 第五远节指骨 fifth distal phalanx

11. 第一指骨粗隆 tuberosity of first phalanx
12. 第一指骨体 shaft of first phalanx
13. 第一指骨底 base of first phalanx
14. 小多角骨 trapezoid
15. 大多角骨 trapezium
16. 头状骨 capitate
17. 手舟骨 scaphoid
18. 钩骨钩 hook of hamate
19. 第一近节指骨滑车 trochlea of first proximal phalanx

图 3-6 右手骨 Bones of right hand
    A. 前面观 Anterior view
    B. 后面观 Posterior view

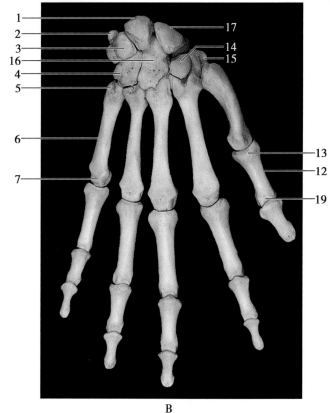

B

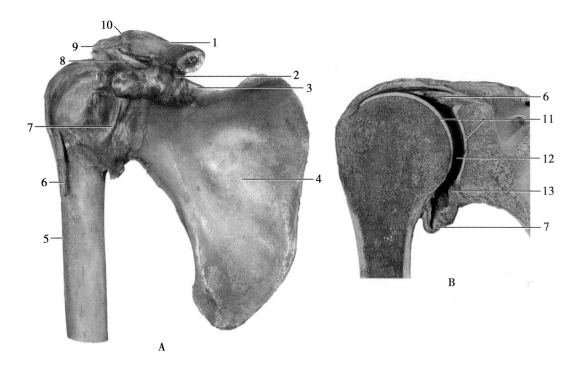

1. 锁骨 clavicle
2. 喙锁韧带 coracoclavicular ligament
3. 肩胛上横韧带 superior transverse scapular ligament
4. 肩胛骨 scapula
5. 肱骨 humerus
6. 肱二头肌长头腱 tendon of long head
   of biceps brachii
7. 关节囊 articular capsule
8. 喙肩韧带 coracoacromial ligament
9. 肩峰 acromion
10. 肩锁关节 acromioclavicular joint
11. 关节软骨 articular cartilage
12. 关节腔 articular cavity
13. 盂唇 glenoid labrum
14. 喙突 coracoid process
15. 关节盂 glenoid cavity

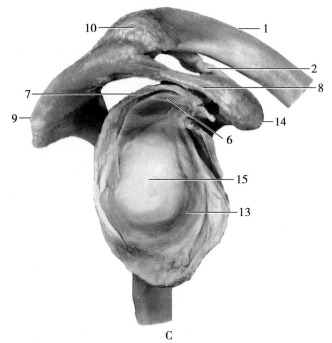

图 3-7　右肩关节 Right shoulder joint
A. 前面观 Anterior view
B. 关节冠状剖面 Frontal section of joint
C. 关节囊已切开 Dissected joint

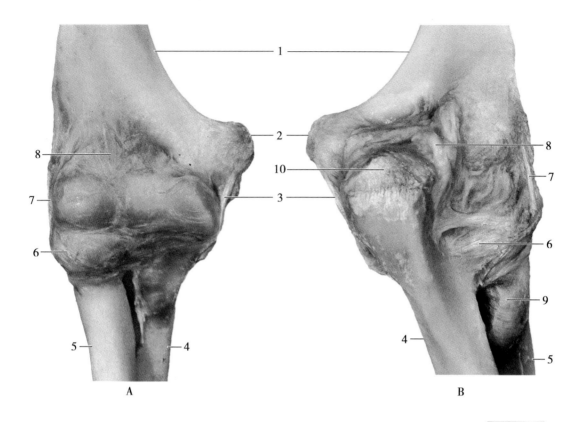

A　　　　　　　　　　　　　　　　　　　B

1. 肱骨 humerus
2. 肱骨内上髁 medial epicondyle of humerus
3. 尺侧副韧带 ulnar collateral ligament
4. 尺骨 ulna
5. 桡骨 radius
6. 桡骨环状韧带 annular ligament of radius
7. 桡侧副韧带 radial collateral ligament
8. 关节囊 articular capsule
9. 桡骨粗隆 radial tuberosity
10. 鹰嘴 olecranon
11. 肱骨滑车 trochlea of humerus
12. 关节腔 articular cavity
13. 肱二头肌腱 tendon of biceps brachii

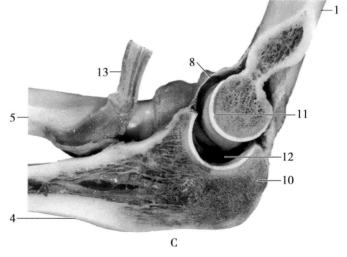

C

图 3-8　右肘关节 Right elbow joint
A. 前面观 Anterior view
B. 后面观 Posterior view
C. 关节矢状剖面 Sagittal Sectioned joint

51

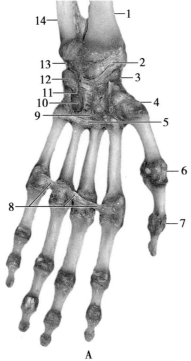

A

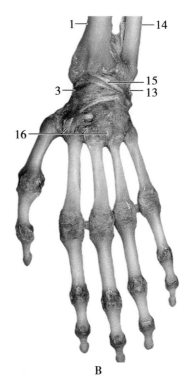

B

1. 桡骨 radius
2. 桡腕掌侧韧带 palmar radiocarpal ligament
3. 腕桡侧副韧带 carporadial collateral ligament
4. 拇指腕掌关节 carpometacarpal joint of thumb
5. 掌骨间韧带 interosseous metacarpal ligament
6. 第一掌指关节 first metacarpophalangeal joint
7. 指间关节 interphalangeal joint
8. 掌骨深横韧带 deep transverse metacarpal ligament
9. 掌侧腕掌韧带 palmar carpometacarpal ligament
10. 钩骨钩 hook of hamate
11. 豆钩韧带 pisohamate ligament
12. 豌豆骨 pisiform
13. 腕尺侧副韧带 carpoulnar collateral ligament
14. 尺骨 ulna
15. 背侧桡腕韧带 dorsal radiocarpal ligament
16. 背侧腕掌韧带 dorsal carpometacarpal ligament
17. 指间关节腔 interphalangeal joint cavity
18. 掌指关节腔 metacarpophalangeal joint cavity
19. 腕掌关节腔 caropmetacarpal joint cavity
20. 腕骨间关节腔 intercarpal joint cavity
21. 关节盘 articular disc
22. 远侧桡尺关节腔 distal radioulnar joint cavity
23. 桡腕关节腔 radiocarpal joint cavity
24. 拇指腕掌关节腔 carpometacarpal joint cavity of thumb

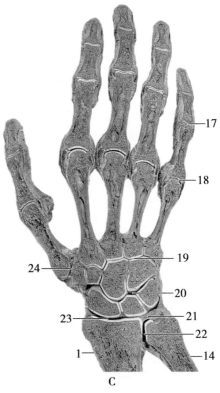

C

图 3-9　左手骨关节 Joints of left hand

A. 前面观 Anterior view　B. 后面观 Posterior view　C. 冠状剖面 Coronal section through joints

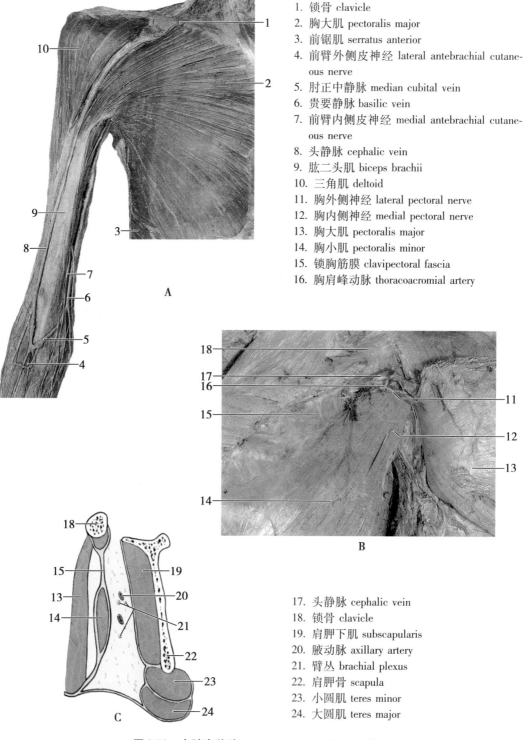

1. 锁骨 clavicle
2. 胸大肌 pectoralis major
3. 前锯肌 serratus anterior
4. 前臂外侧皮神经 lateral antebrachial cutaneous nerve
5. 肘正中静脉 median cubital vein
6. 贵要静脉 basilic vein
7. 前臂内侧皮神经 medial antebrachial cutaneous nerve
8. 头静脉 cephalic vein
9. 肱二头肌 biceps brachii
10. 三角肌 deltoid
11. 胸外侧神经 lateral pectoral nerve
12. 胸内侧神经 medial pectoral nerve
13. 胸大肌 pectoralis major
14. 胸小肌 pectoralis minor
15. 锁胸筋膜 clavipectoral fascia
16. 胸肩峰动脉 thoracoacromial artery

17. 头静脉 cephalic vein
18. 锁骨 clavicle
19. 肩胛下肌 subscapularis
20. 腋动脉 axillary artery
21. 臂丛 brachial plexus
22. 肩胛骨 scapula
23. 小圆肌 teres minor
24. 大圆肌 teres major

图 3-10 右腋窝前壁 Anterior wall of right axilla
A. 胸大肌（前面观）Pectoralis major（anterior view）
B. 胸小肌（前面观）Pectoralis minor（anterior view）
C. 矢状剖面示意图 Diagram for sagittal section through axilla

53

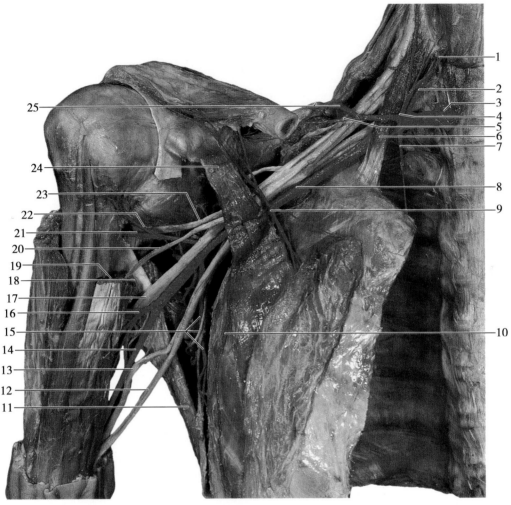

图 3-11　右腋窝内神经血管（前面观）
Nerves and blood vessels in right axilla（anterior view）
保留胸小肌 Pectoralis minor been kept

1. 甲状腺下动脉 inferior thyroid artery
2. 椎动脉 vertebral artery
3. 锁骨下动脉 subclavian artery
4. 甲状颈干 thyrocervical trunk
5. 肩胛上动脉 suprascapular artery
6. 前斜角肌 scalenus anterior
7. 胸廓内动脉 internal thoracic artery
8. 腋动脉 axillary artery
9. 胸肩峰动脉 thoracoacromial artery
10. 胸外侧动脉 lateral thoracic artery
11. 背阔肌 latissimus dorsi
12. 正中神经 median nerve
13. 尺神经 ulnar nerve
14. 肱动脉 brachial artery
15. 胸背动脉和胸背神经 thoracodorsal artery and nerve
16. 肱深动脉 deep brachial artery
17. 桡神经 radial nerve
18. 喙肱肌 coracobrachialis
19. 肱二头肌 biceps brachii
20. 肌皮神经 musculocutaneous nerve
21. 旋肱后动脉 posterior circumflex humeral artery
22. 旋肱前动脉 anterior circumflex humeral artery
23. 腋神经 axillary nerve
24. 胸小肌 pectoralis minor
25. 颈浅动脉与肩胛提肌 superficial cervical artery and levator scapulae

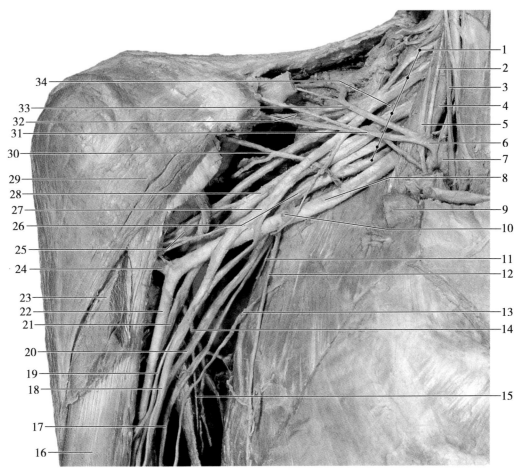

图 3-12　右腋窝内臂丛和血管(前面观)
Nerves and blood vessels in right axilla(anterior view)
前壁完全去除 Anterior wall been completely removed

1. 臂丛的 5 条根 5 roots of brachial plexus
2. 颈升动脉 ascending cervical artery
3. 迷走神经 vagus nerve
4. 前斜角肌 scalenus anterior
5. 膈神经 phrenic nerve
6. 甲状颈干 thyrocervical trunk
7. 锁骨下动脉 subclavian artery
8. 腋动脉 axillary artery
9. 锁骨下静脉 subclavian vein
10. 胸肩峰动脉 thoracoacromial artery
11. 胸长神经 long thoracic nerve
12. 胸外侧动脉 lateral thoracic artery
13. 肋间臂神经 intercostobrachial nerve
14. 胸背动脉 thoracodorsal artery
15. 胸背神经 thoracodorsal nerve
16. 肱二头肌 biceps brachii
17. 前臂内侧皮神经 medial antebrachial cutaneous nerve

18. 正中神经 median nerve
19. 肌皮神经 musculocutaneous nerve
20. 尺神经 ulnar nerve
21. 桡神经 radial nerve
22. 肱动脉 brachial artery
23. 胸大肌 pectoralis major
24. 旋肱后动脉 posterior circumflex humeral artery
25. 腋神经 axillary nerve
26. 臂丛内侧束 medial cord of brachial plexus
27. 臂丛外侧束 lateral cord of brachial plexus
28. 臂丛后束 posterior cord of brachial plexus
29. 三角肌 deltoid
30. 腋动脉三角肌支 deltoid branch of axillary artery
31. 肩胛上动脉 suprascapular artery
32. 肩胛上神经 suprascapular nerve
33. 颈横动脉 transverse cervical artery
34. 中斜角肌 scalenum medius

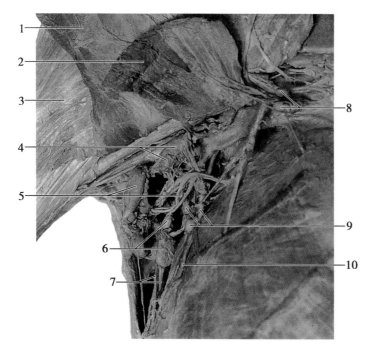

图 3-13　右腋淋巴结（前面观）
Lymph nodes in right axilla
（anterior view）

1. 胸大肌 pectoralis major
2. 胸小肌 pectoralis minor
3. 三角肌 deltoid
4. 外侧淋巴结 lateral lymph nodes
5. 中央淋巴结 central lymph nodes
6. 肩胛下淋巴结 subscapular lymph nodes
7. 胸背动脉和神经 thoracodorsal artery and nerve
8. 尖淋巴结 apical lymph nodes
9. 胸肌淋巴结 pectoral lymph nodes
10. 胸外侧动脉 lateral thoracic artery

图 3-14　右臂前面肌、神经和血管（前面观）
Muscles，nerves and blood vessels in anterior
compartment of upper arm（anterior view）

1. 三角肌 deltoid
2. 胸大肌 pectoralis major
3. 腋神经 axillary nerve
4. 肌皮神经 musculocutaneous nerve
5. 肱二头肌短头 short head of biceps brachii
6. 肱二头肌长头 long head of biceps brachii
7. 尺神经 ulnar nerve
8. 正中神经 median nerve
9. 前臂外侧皮神经 lateral antebrachial cutaneous nerve
10. 肱二头肌腱膜 bicipital aponeurosis
11. 锁骨 clavicle
12. 胸小肌 pectoralis minor
13. 腋动脉 axillary artery
14. 桡神经 radial nerve
15. 胸外侧动脉 lateral thoracic artery
16. 胸背动脉 thoracodorsal artery

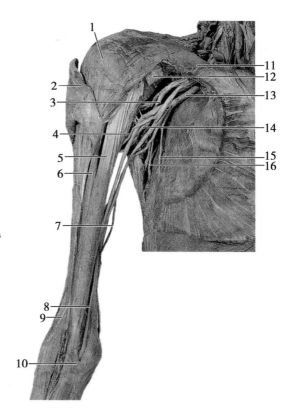

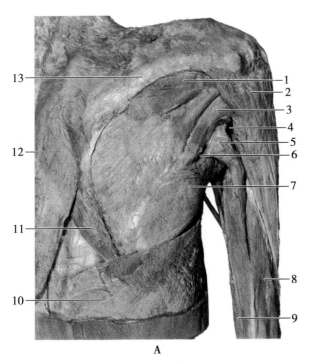

A

1. 冈下肌 infraspinatus
2. 三角肌 deltoid
3. 小圆肌 teres minor
4. 四边孔 quadrangular space
5. 肱三头肌长头 long head of triceps brachii
6. 三边孔 triangular space
7. 大圆肌 teres major
8. 肱三头肌外侧头 lateral head of triceps brachii
9. 肱三头肌内侧头 medial head of triceps brachii
10. 背阔肌 latissimus dorsi
11. 菱形肌 rhomboid
12. 斜方肌 trapezius

13. 肩胛冈 spine of scapula
14. 腋神经和旋肱后动脉 axillary nerve and posterior circumflex humeral artery
15. 旋肩胛动脉 circumflex scapular artery
16. 肱深动脉 deep brachial artery
17. 前臂后皮神经 posterior cutaneous nerve of the forearm
18. 桡神经 radial nerve
19. 桡侧副动脉 radial collateral artery
20. 中副动脉 middle collateral artery
21. 桡神经后肌支 posterior muscular branch of radial nerve
22. 冈上肌 supraspinatus

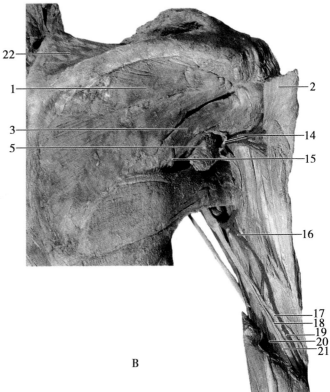

B

图 3-15　右肩胛区和臂后区的结构(后面观)
Structures of right scapular and posterior brachial regions(posterior view)
A. 肌 Muscles　B. 腋神经和桡神经 Axillary nerve and radial nerve

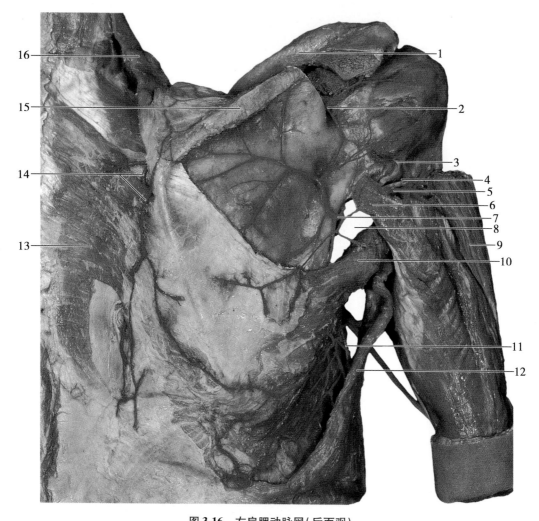

图 3-16 右肩胛动脉网(后面观)
Right scapular anastomosis(posterior view)

1. 锁骨 clavicle
2. 肩胛上动脉 suprascapular artery
3. 腋神经 axillary nerve
4. 四边孔 quadrangular space
5. 旋肱后动脉 posterior circumflex humeral artery
6. 肱三头肌长头 long head of triceps brachii
7. 旋肩胛动脉 circumflex scapular artery
8. 三边孔 triangular space

9. 三角肌 deltoid
10. 大圆肌 teres major
11. 胸背神经 thoracodorsal nerve
12. 背阔肌 latissimus dorsi
13. 菱形肌 rhomboid
14. 肩胛背动脉 dorsal scapular artery
15. 肩胛冈 spine of scapula
16. 肩胛提肌 levator scapulae

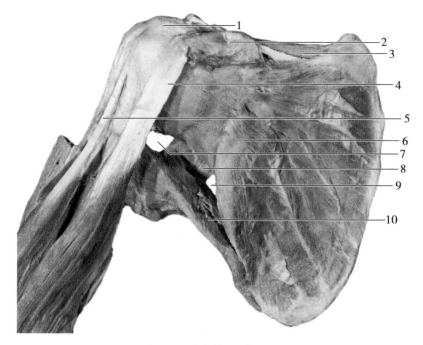

图 3-17　右肩袖肌（前面观）
Right rotator cuff（anterior view）

1. 肩关节囊 articular capsule of should joint
2. 喙突 coracoid process
3. 冈上肌 suparspinatus
4. 肱二头肌短头 short head of biceps brachii
5. 肱二头肌长头 long head of biceps brachii
6. 肩胛下肌 subscapularis
7. 四边孔 quadrangular space
8. 肱三头肌长头 long head of triceps brachii
9. 三边孔 triangular space
10. 大圆肌 teres major

1. 冈上肌 srpraspinatus
2. 肩关节囊 articular capsule of should joint
3. 肩胛冈 spine of scapula
4. 冈下肌 infraspinatus
5. 小圆肌 teres minor
6. 四边孔 quadrangular space
7. 肱三头肌长头 long head of triceps brachii
8. 三边孔 triangular space
9. 大圆肌 teres major
10. 三角肌 deltoid

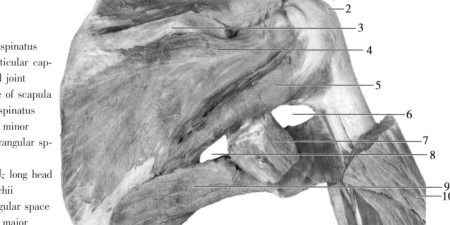

图 3-18　右肩袖肌（后面观）
Right rotator cuff（posterior view）

59

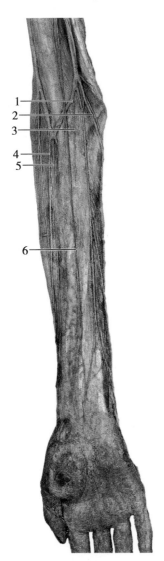

1. 正中神经 median nerve
2. 旋前圆肌 pronator teres
3. 掌长肌 palmaris longus
4. 指浅屈肌 flexor digitorum superficialis
5. 尺侧腕屈肌 flexor carpi ulnaris
6. 尺动脉和尺静脉 ulnar artery and vein
7. 掌短肌 palmaris brevis
8. 掌腱膜 palmar aponeurosis
9. 拇短展肌 abductor pollicis brevis
10. 正中神经 median nerve
11. 桡动脉和静脉 radial artery and vein
12. 桡侧腕屈肌 flexor carpi radialis
13. 肱桡肌 brachioradialis
14. 前臂外侧皮神经 lateral antebrachial cutaneous nerve
15. 肱动脉 brachial artery
16. 肱二头肌 biceps brachii

图 3-19　右肘窝和前臂皮神经和浅静脉（前面观）
Cutaneous nerves and superficial veins on right cubital region and forearm（anterior view）

1. 肘正中静脉 median cubital vein
2. 贵要静脉 basilic vein
3. 前臂正中静脉 median antebrachial vein
4. 头静脉 cephalic vein
5. 前臂外侧皮神经 lateral antebrachial cutaneous nerve
6. 前臂内侧皮神经 medial antebrachial cutaneous nerve

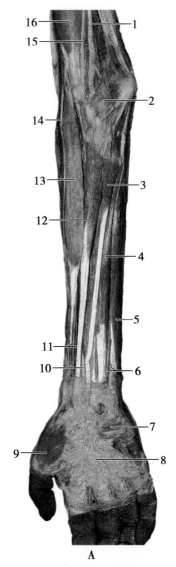

A

图 3-20　右前臂前区的肌（前面观）
Muscles in anterior compartment of right forearm（anterior view）

A. 第 1 层 First layer

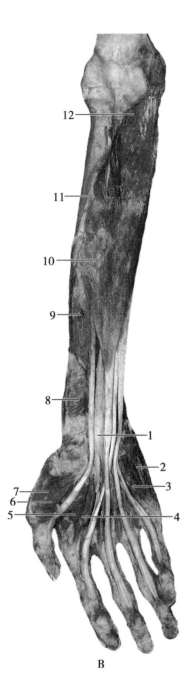

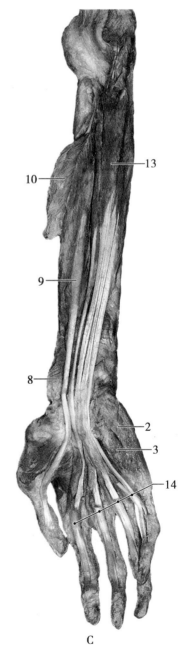

图 3-20　右前臂前区的肌(前面观)(续)
Muscles in anterior compartment of right forearm(anterior view)(continued)
　　　B. 第 2 层 Second layer
　　　C. 第 3 层 Third layer

1. 指深屈肌腱 tendon of flexor digitorum profundus
2. 小指展肌 abductor digiti minimi
3. 小指短屈肌 flexor digiti minimi brevis
4. 蚓状肌 lumbricals
5. 拇收肌 adductor pollicis

6. 拇短屈肌 flexor pollicis brevis
7. 拇对掌肌 opponens pollicis
8. 旋前方肌 pronator quadatus
9. 拇长屈肌 flexor pollicis longus
10. 指浅屈肌 flexor digitorum superficialis
11. 指浅屈肌桡头 radial head of flexor digitorum superficialis
12. 指浅屈肌肱尺头 humeroulnar head of flexor digitorum superficialis
13. 指深屈肌 flexor digitorum profundus
14. 指浅屈肌腱 tendon of flexor digitorum superficialis

61

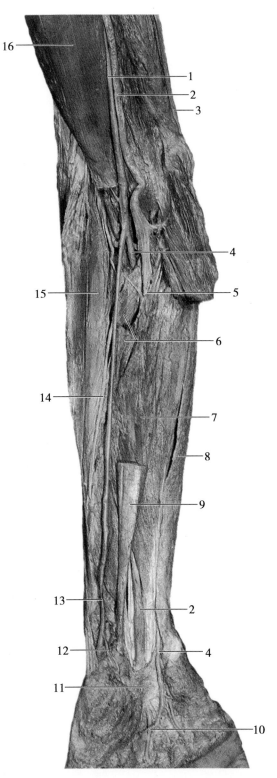

1. 肱动脉 brachial artery
2. 正中神经 median nerve
3. 尺神经 ulnar nerve
4. 尺动脉 ulnar artery
5. 指浅屈肌腱弓 tendinous arch of flexor digitorum superficialis
6. 旋前圆肌 pronator teres
7. 指浅屈肌 flexor digitorum superficialis
8. 尺侧腕屈肌 flexor carpi ulnaris
9. 桡侧腕屈肌 flexor carpi radialis
10. 掌浅弓 superficial palmar arch
11. 屈肌支持带 flexor retinaculum
12. 掌浅支 superficial palmar branch of radial artery
13. 桡动脉 radial artery
14. 桡神经浅支 superficial branch of radial nerve
15. 肱桡肌 brachioradialis
16. 肱二头肌 biceps brachii

图 3-21　右肘窝内神经血管（前面观）
Nerves and blood vessels in right cubital fossa
（anterior view）

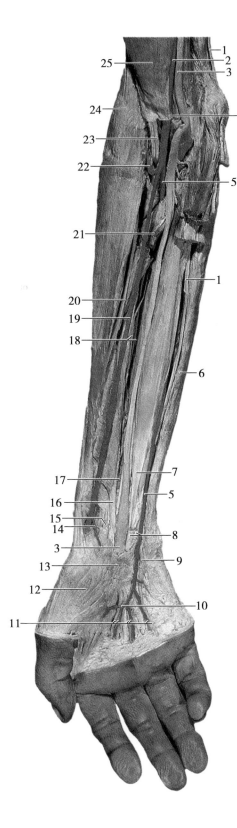

1. 尺神经 ulnar nerve
2. 肱动脉 brachial artery
3. 正中神经 median nerve
4. 肱二头肌腱膜 bicipital aponeurosis
5. 尺动脉 ulnar artery
6. 尺侧腕屈肌 flexor carpi ulnaris
7. 指深屈肌 flexor digitorum profundus
8. 指浅屈肌腱 tendon of flexor digitorum superficialis
9. 尺神经浅支 superficial branch of ulnar nerve
10. 掌浅弓 superficial palmar arch
11. 指掌侧总动脉及神经 common palmar digital artery and nerve
12. 拇短展肌 abductor pollicis brevis
13. 屈肌支持带 flexor retinaculum
14. 桡动脉掌浅支 superficial palmar branch of radial artery
15. 桡侧腕屈肌腱 tendon of flexor carpi radialis
16. 拇长屈肌腱 tendon of flexor pollicis longus
17. 旋前方肌 pronator quadratus
18. 骨间前动脉和神经 anterior interosseus artery and nerve
19. 桡动脉 radial artery
20. 桡神经浅支 superficial branch of radial nerve
21. 旋前圆肌 pronator teres
22. 桡侧返动脉 radial recurrent artery
23. 肱二头肌腱 tendon of biceps brachii
24. 肱桡肌 brachioradialis
25. 肱二头肌 biceps brachii

图 3-22　右前臂前区的神经血管（前面观）
Nerves and blood vessels in anterior compartment of right forearm（anterior view）

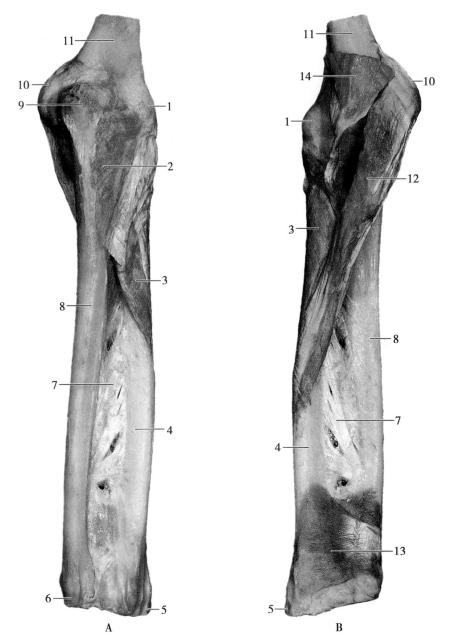

A　　　　　　　　　　　　　B

图 3-23　右前臂旋前肌和旋后肌
Muscles for pronation and supination of right forearm
A. 后面观 Posterior view　B. 前面观 Anterior view

1. 肱骨外上髁 lateral epicondyle of humerus
2. 肘肌 anconeus
3. 旋后肌 supinator
4. 桡骨 radius
5. 桡骨茎突 styloid process of radius
6. 尺骨茎突 styloid process of ulna
7. 前臂骨间膜 interosseous membrane of forearm

8. 尺骨 ulnar
9. 鹰嘴 olecranon
10. 肱骨内上髁 medial epicondyle of humerus
11. 肱骨 humerus
12. 旋前圆肌 pronator teres
13. 旋前方肌 pronator quadratus
14. 肱二头肌 biceps brachii

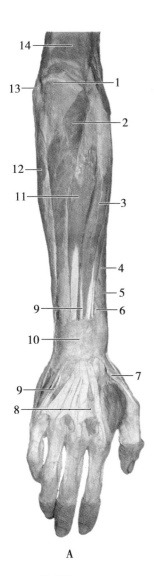

A

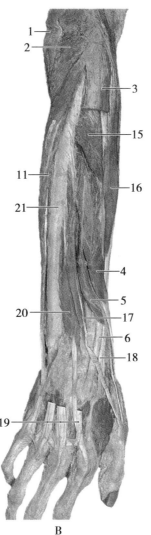

B

图 3-25　右前臂后区神经血管(后面观)
Nerves and blood vessels in posterior compartment of right forearm(posterior view)

图 3-24　右前臂后区肌(后面观)
Muscles in posterior compartment of right forearm(posterior view)

　　A. 浅层 Superficial layer
　　B. 深层 Deep layer

1. 鹰嘴 olecranon
2. 肘肌 anconeus
3. 指伸肌 extensor digitorum
4. 拇长展肌 abductor pollicis longus
5. 拇短伸肌 extensor pollicis brevis
6. 桡侧腕短伸肌腱 tendon of extensor carpi radialis brevis
7. 拇长伸肌腱 tendon of extensor pollicis longus
8. 腱间结合 intertendinous connection
9. 小指伸肌 extensor digiti minimi
10. 伸肌支持带 extensor retinaculum
11. 尺侧腕伸肌 extensor carpi ulnaris
12. 尺侧腕屈肌 flexor carpi ulnaris
13. 尺神经 ulnar nerve
14. 肱三头肌 triceps brachii

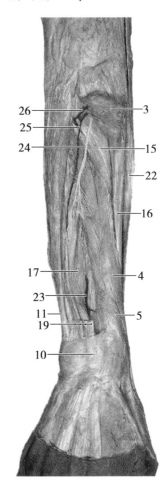

15. 旋后肌 supinator
16. 桡侧腕短伸肌 extensor carpi radialis brevis
17. 拇长伸肌 extensor pollicis longus
18. 桡侧腕长伸肌腱 tendon of extensor carpi radialis longus
19. 指伸肌腱 tendon of extensor digitorum
20. 示指伸肌 extensor indicis
21. 尺骨 ulnar
22. 桡侧腕长伸肌 extensor carpi radialis longus
23. 骨间前动脉后支 posterior branch of anterior interosseous artery
24. 骨间后神经 posterior interosseous nerve
25. 骨间后动脉 posterior interosseous artery
26. 骨间返动脉 recurrent interosseous artery

65

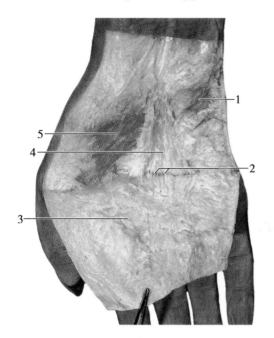

图 3-26　右手掌腱膜（前面观）
Palmar aponeurosis of right hand（anterior view）
1. 掌短肌 palmaris brevis
2. 纤维隔 fibrous septa
3. 皮肤与浅筋膜 skin and superficial fascia
4. 掌腱膜 palmar aponeurosis
5. 鱼际肌 thenar muscles

图 3-27　右手掌浅弓和神经（前面观）
Superficial palmar arch and nerves of right hand（anterior view）

1. 贵要静脉 basilic vein
2. 尺侧腕屈肌腱 tendon of flexor carpi ulnaris
3. 尺动脉 ulnar artery
4. 指浅屈肌腱 tendon of flexor digitorum superficialis
5. 尺神经深支及尺动脉掌深支 deep branch of ulnar nerve and deep palmar branch of ulnar artery
6. 尺神经浅支 superficial branch of ulnar nerve
7. 掌浅弓 superficial palmar arch
8. 指掌侧总神经 common palmar digital nerve
9. 小指尺掌侧固有动脉及神经 ulnar palmar artery and nerve of little finger
10. 指掌侧总动脉 common palmar digital artery
11. 指掌侧固有动脉及神经 proper palmar digital artery and nerve
12. 蚓状肌 lumbricals
13. 拇短屈肌 flexor pollicis brevis
14. 正中神经返支 recurrent branch of median nerve
15. 桡动脉掌浅支 superficial palmar branch of radial artery
16. 拇短展肌 abductor pollicis brevis
17. 屈肌支持带 flexor retinaculum
18. 正中神经 median nerve
19. 桡侧腕屈肌腱 tendon of flexor carpi radialis
20. 桡动脉 radial artery

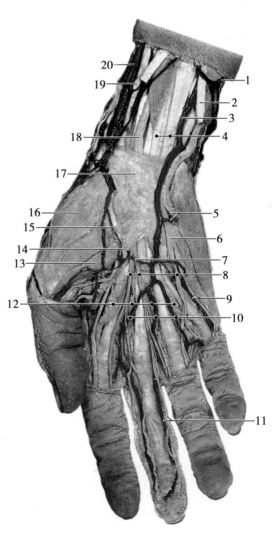

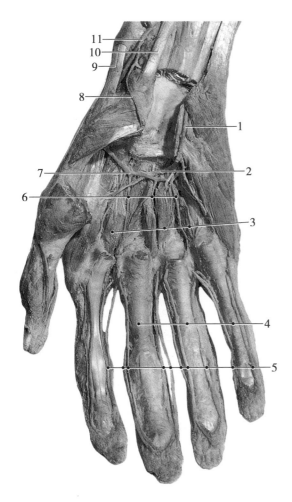

图 3-29 右手屈指肌腱和滑膜鞘(前面观)
Flexor tendons and synovial sheaths of right hand (anterior view)

1. 尺侧腕屈肌 flexor carpi ulnaris
2. 屈肌总腱鞘 common flexor synovial sheath
3. 小指展肌 abductor digiti minimi
4. 小指短屈肌 flexor digiti minimi brevis
5. 蚓状肌 lumbricals
6. 小指指浅屈肌和指深屈肌腱鞘 synovial sheath for tendons of flexor digitorum superficialis and profundus of little finger
7. 示指、中指和环指指浅屈肌和指深屈肌腱鞘 synovial sheath for tendons of flexor digitorum superficialis and profundus of index，middle and ring fingers
8. 拇长屈肌腱鞘 synovial sheath for tendon of flexor pollicis longus
9. 拇收肌 adductor pollicis
10. 拇短屈肌 flexor pollicis brevis
11. 拇短展肌 abductor pollicis brevis
12. 掌长肌腱 tendon of palmaris longus

图 3-28 右手掌深弓和神经(前面观)
Deep palmar arch and nerves of right hand (anterior view)

1. 尺动脉 ulnar artery
2. 尺神经深支 deep branch of ulnar nerve
3. 骨间掌侧肌 palmar interossei
4. 腱纤维鞘 fibrous digital sheaths
5. 指掌侧固有动脉及神经 proper palmar digital artery and nerve
6. 掌心动脉 palmar metacarpal artery
7. 掌深弓 deep palmar arch
8. 桡动脉掌浅支 superficial palmar branch of radial artery
9. 肱桡肌腱 tendon of brachioradialis
10. 桡侧腕屈肌腱 tendon of flexor carpi radialis
11. 桡动脉 radial artery

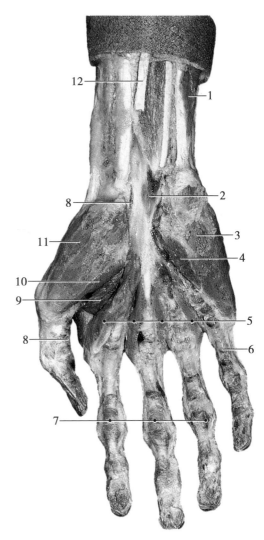

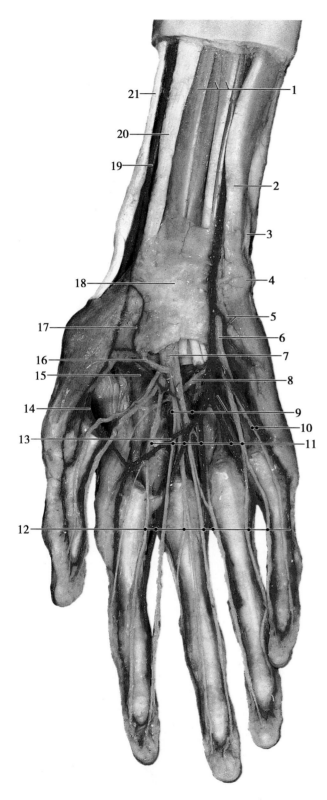

1. 指浅屈肌 flexor digitorum superficialis
2. 尺侧腕屈肌腱 tendon of flexor carpi ulnaris
3. 尺神经背支 dorsal branch of ulnar nerve
4. 豌豆骨 pisiform
5. 尺动脉掌深支及尺神经深支 deep palmar branch of ulnar artery and deep branch of ulnar nerve
6. 尺神经浅支 superficial branch of ulnar nerve
7. 正中神经 median nerve
8. 尺神经深支 deep branch of ulnar nerve
9. 掌心动脉 palmar metacarpal arteries
10. 小指尺掌侧动脉及神经 ulnar palmar artery and nerve of little finger
11. 指掌侧总动脉及神经 common palmar digital arteries and nerves
12. 指掌侧固有动脉和神经 proper palmar digital arteries and nerves
13. 掌浅弓 superficial palmar arch
14. 拇主要动脉 princeps pollicis artery
15. 掌深弓 deep palmar arch
16. 正中神经返支 recurrent branch of median nerve
17. 桡动脉掌浅支 superficial palmar branch of radial artery
18. 屈肌支持带 flexor retinaculum
19. 桡动脉 radial artery
20. 桡侧腕屈肌腱 tendon of flexor carpi radialis
21. 肱桡肌腱 tendon of brachioradialis

图 3-30 右手腕部神经血管(前面观)
Nerves and blood vessels of right wrist and hand(anterior view)

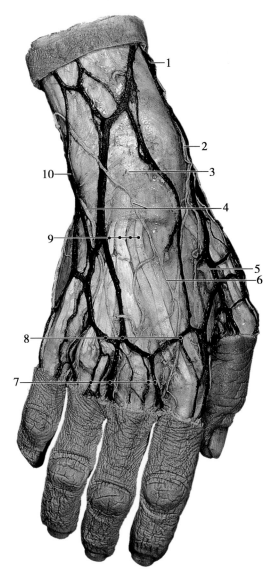

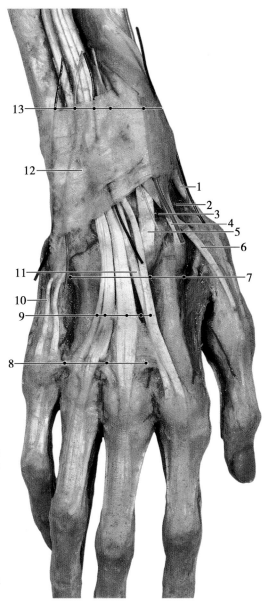

图 3-31 右手腕部皮神经和浅静脉(后面观)
Cutaneous nerves and superficial veins of
right wrist and hand(posterior view)

1. 头静脉 cephalic vein
2. 桡神经浅支 superficial branch of radial nerve
3. 伸肌支持带 extensor retinaculum
4. 尺神经手背支 dorsal branches of ulnar nerve
5. 第一掌背动脉 first dorsal metacarpal artery
6. 尺神经交通支 communicating branch of ulnar nerve
7. 指背静脉网 dorsal venous rete of fingers
8. 手背静脉网 dorsal venous network
9. 指伸肌腱 tendons of extensor digitorum
10. 贵要静脉 basilic vein

图 3-32 右手背伸肌腱和动脉(后面观)
Extensor tendons and arteries on dorsal aspect of
right wrist and hand(posterior view)

1. 拇短伸肌腱 tendon of extensor pollicis brevis
2. 桡动脉 radial artery
3. 桡动脉腕背支 dorsal carpal branch of radial artery
4. 桡侧腕长伸肌腱 tendon of extensor carpi radialis longus
5. 桡侧腕短伸肌腱 tendon of extensor carpi radialis brevis
6. 拇长伸肌腱 tendon of extensor pollicis longus
7. 掌背动脉 dorsal palmar artery
8. 腱间结合 intertendinous connections
9. 指伸肌腱 tendons of extensor digitorum
10. 小指伸肌腱 tendon of extensor digiti minimi
11. 示指伸肌腱 tendon of extensor indicis
12. 伸肌支持带 extensor retinaculum
13. 腕背骨纤维管 osseofibrous canal of posterior region
   of wrist

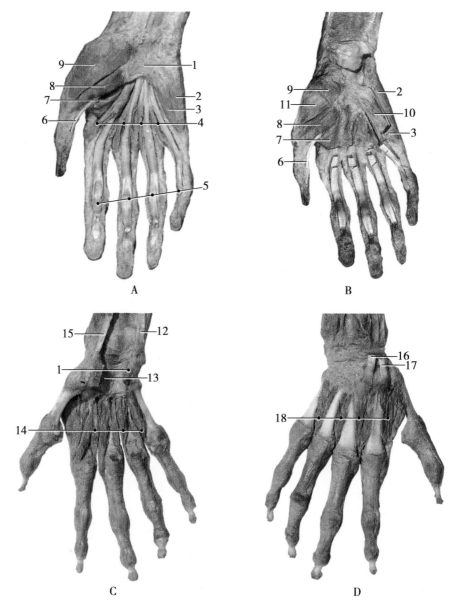

A

B

C

D

图 3-33　右手肌 Muscles of right hand

A. 前面观 Anterior view　B. 鱼际肌和小鱼际肌 Thenar muscles and hypothenar muscles

C. 骨间掌侧肌 Palmar interossei　D. 后面观 Posterior view

1. 屈肌支持带 flexor retinaculum
2. 小指展肌 abductor digiti minimi
3. 小指短屈肌 flexor digiti minimi brevis
4. 蚓状肌 lumbricals
5. 指深屈肌腱 tendon of flexor digitorum profundus
6. 拇长屈肌腱 tendon of flexor pollicis longus
7. 拇收肌 adductor pollicis
8. 拇短屈肌 flexor pollicis brevis
9. 拇短展肌 abductor pollicis brevis
10. 小指对掌肌 opponens digiti minimi

11. 拇对掌肌 opponens pollicis
12. 尺侧腕屈肌腱 tendon of flexor carpi ulnaris
13. 腕管 carpal canal
14. 骨间掌侧肌 palmar interossei
15. 桡侧腕屈肌腱 tendon of flexor carpi radialis
16. 桡侧腕短伸肌腱 tendon of extensor carpi radialis brevis
17. 桡侧腕长伸肌腱 tendon of extensor carpi radialis longus
18. 骨间背侧肌 dorsal interossei

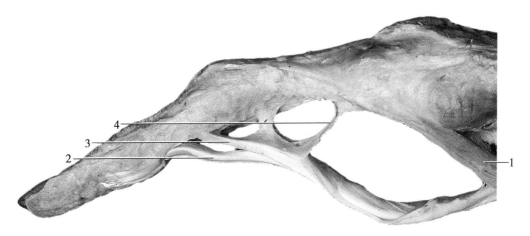

图 3-34　右示指屈肌腱和腱纽(外侧观)
Flexor tendons and vincula tendinum of index finger of right hand(lateral view)

1. 蚓状肌 lumbricals
2. 指深屈肌腱 tendon of flexor digitorum profundus
3. 指浅屈肌腱 tendon of flexor digitorum superficialis
4. 腱纽 vincula tendinum

1. 正中神经 median nerve
2. 贵要静脉 basilic vein
3. 肱动脉及静脉 brachial artery and vein
4. 尺神经与尺侧上副动脉 ulnar nerve and superior ulnar collateral artery
5. 肱三头肌内侧头 medial head of triceps brachii
6. 肱三头肌长头 long head of triceps brachii
7. 肱三头肌外侧头 lateral head of triceps brachii
8. 桡神经 radial nerve
9. 肱深动脉及静脉 deep brachial artery and vein
10. 肱肌 brachialis
11. 肌皮神经 musculocutaneous nerve
12. 头静脉 cephalic vein
13. 肱二头肌 biceps brachii

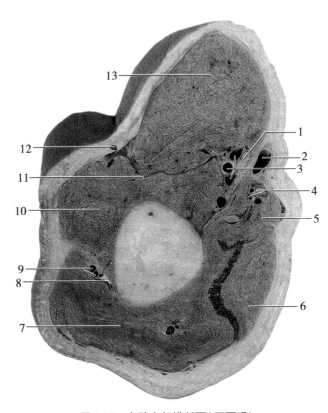

图 3-35　右臂中部横断面(下面观)
Transverse section through middle of right upper arm(inferior view)

71

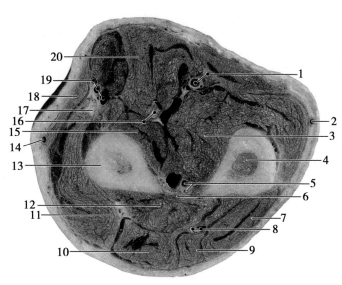

图 3-36 右前臂中部横断面(下面观)
Transverse section through middle of right forearm(inferior view)

1. 尺神经及动脉 ulnar nerve and artery
2. 贵要静脉 basilic vein
3. 指深屈肌 flexor digitorum profundus
4. 尺骨 ulna
5. 骨间前动脉及静脉 anterior interosse- ous artery and vein
6. 前臂骨间膜 interosseous membrane of forearm
7. 尺侧腕伸肌 extensor carpi ulnaris
8. 骨间后动脉及静脉 posterior interosse- ous artery and vein
9. 小指伸肌 extensor digiti minimi
10. 指伸肌 extensor digitorum
11. 桡侧腕短伸肌 extensor carpi radia- lis brevis
12. 旋后肌 supinator
13. 桡骨 radius
14. 头静脉 cephalic vein
15. 拇长屈肌 flexor pollicis longus
16. 正中神经 median nerve
17. 桡神经 radial nerve
18. 肱桡肌 brachioradialis
19. 桡动脉及静脉 radial artery and vein
20. 指浅屈肌 flexor digitorum superfi- cialis

1. 拇短展肌 abductor pollicis brevis
2. 掌腱膜 palmar aponeurosis
3. 拇长屈肌腱 tendon of flex- or pollicis longus
4. 蚓状肌 lumbricals
5. 掌中隔 midpalmar septum
6. 拇收肌 adductor pollicis
7. 掌深弓 deep palmar arch
8. 骨间背侧肌 dorsal interos- sei
9. 骨间掌侧肌 palmar interos- sei
10. 第五掌骨 fifth metacarpal
11. 掌中间隙 midpalmar space
12. 指深屈肌腱 tendons of flexor digitorum profundus
13. 指浅屈肌腱 tendons of flexor digitorum surperfi- cialis
14. 正中神经分支 branches of median nerve
15. 尺神经浅支 superficial branch of ulnar nerve
16. 小指展肌 abductor digiti minimi
17. 尺动脉及静脉 ulnar ar- tery and vein

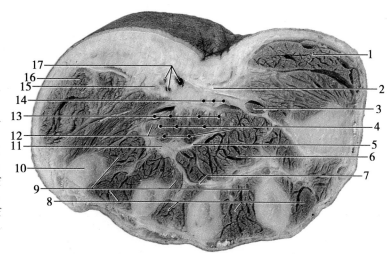

图 3-37 右手掌横断面(下面观)
Transverse section through metacarpals of right hand(inferior view)

第 4 章　胸

Chapter 4　Thorax

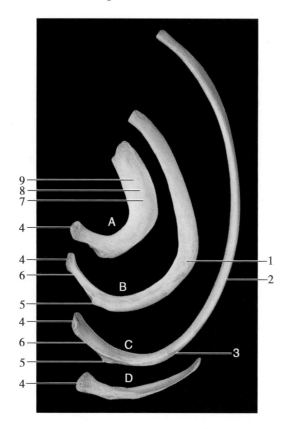

图 4-1 左侧肋骨（上面观）
Left ribs（superior view）

A. 第一肋 first rib　B. 第二肋 second rib　C. 第
　　六肋 sixth rib　D. 第十二肋 twelfth rib

1. 前锯肌粗隆 tuberosity for serratus anterior
2. 肋体 body of rib
3. 肋角 angle of rib
4. 肋头 head of rib
5. 肋结节 tubercle of rib
6. 肋颈 neck of rib
7. 锁骨下动脉沟 groove for subclavian artery
8. 斜角肌结节 scalene tubercle
9. 锁骨下静脉沟 groove for subclavian vein

图 4-2 胸骨 Sternum
A. 前面观 Anterior view　B. 右侧面观
　　Right lateral view

1. 胸骨角 sternal angle
2. 第三肋切迹 third costal notch
3. 第四肋切迹 fourth costal notch
4. 第五肋切迹 fifth costal notch
5. 第六、第七肋切迹 sixth and seventh
　　costal notch
6. 锁切迹 clavicular notch
7. 第一肋切迹 first costal notch
8. 胸骨柄 manubrium
9. 第二肋切迹 second costal notch
10. 胸骨体 body of sternum
11. 剑突 xiphoid process
12. 颈静脉切迹 jugular notch

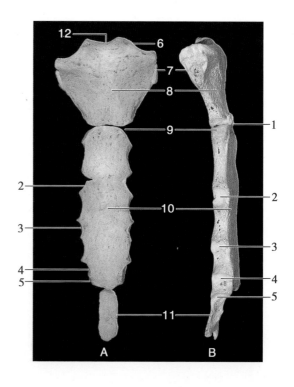

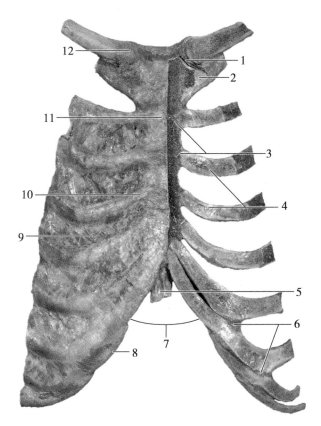

图 4-3　肋与胸骨连接(前面观)
Joints of ribs and sternum
(anterior view)
1. 胸锁关节关节盘 articular disc
   of sternoclavicular joint
2. 第一胸肋结合 first sternocostal joint
3. 第二、第三胸肋关节 second and third
   sternocostal joints
4. 肋软骨 costal cartilages
5. 剑突 xiphoid process
6. 软骨间关节 interchondral joints
7. 胸骨下角 infrasternal angle
8. 肋弓 costal arch
9. 肋间隙 intercostal space
10. 胸肋辐状韧带 radiate sternocostal
    ligament
11. 胸骨角 sternal angle
12. 胸锁关节 sternoclavicular joint

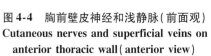
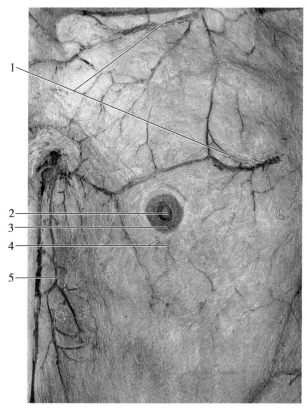

图 4-4　胸前壁皮神经和浅静脉(前面观)
Cutaneous nerves and superficial veins on
anterior thoracic wall(anterior view)
1. 肋间神经穿支 perforating branch of
   intercostal nerve
2. 乳头 mammary papilla
3. 乳晕 areola of breast
4. 乳晕静脉丛 areola venous plexus
5. 胸腹壁静脉 thoracoepigastric vein

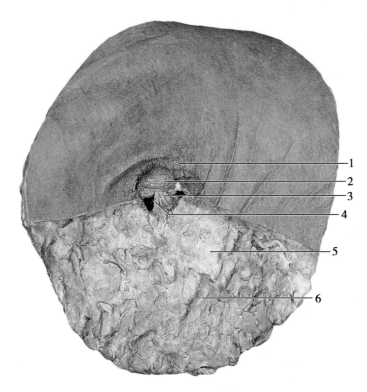

图 4-5　女性乳房（前面观）
Female breast (anterior view)

1. 乳晕 areola of breast
2. 乳头 mammary papilla
3. 输乳管 lactiferous ducts
4. 输乳管窦 lactiferous sinus
5. 脂肪 fat
6. 乳腺小叶 lobules of mammary gland

图 4-6　胸前壁（内面观）
**Anterior wall of thorax
(internal view)**

1. 胸骨舌骨肌 sternohyoid
2. 右锁骨下动脉 right subclavian artery
3. 胸骨甲状肌 sternothyroid
4. 右头臂静脉 right brachiocephalic vein
5. 胸廓内动脉 internal thoracic artery
6. 胸廓内静脉 internal thoracic vein
7. 胸廓内动脉穿支 perforating branch of internal thoracic artery
8. 胸骨旁淋巴结 parasternal lymph nodes
9. 胸膜前反折线 anterior line of pleural reflection
10. 胸横肌 transversus thoracis

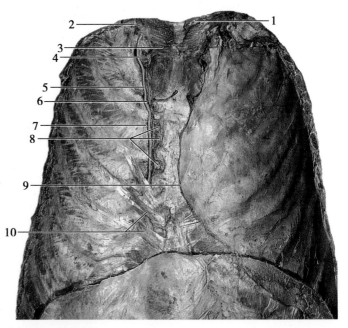

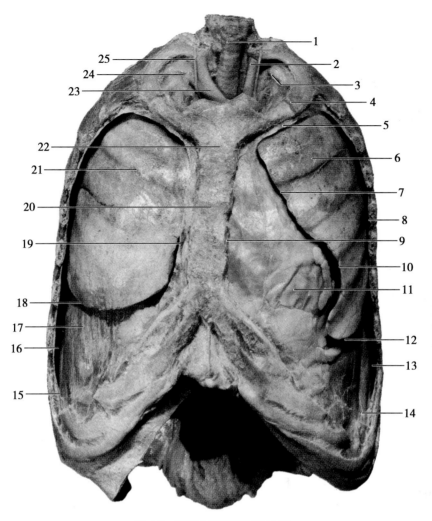

图 4-7　胸膜与胸膜腔（前面观）
Pleura and pleural cavity（anterior view）

1. 气管 trachea
2. 左颈总动脉 left common carotid artery
3. 左肺尖 apex of left lung
4. 第一肋 first rib
5. 肋胸膜 costal pleura
6. 左肺及肺胸膜 left lung and pulmonary pleura
7. 左肺前缘 anterior margin of left lung
8. 胸膜腔 pleural cavity
9. 左肋纵隔胸膜返折线 left costomediastinal line of pleural reflection
10. 心切迹 cardiac notch of left lung
11. 心包及纵隔胸膜 pericardium and mediastinal pleura
12. 左肺下缘 inferior margin of left lung
13. 左肋膈隐窝 left costodiaphragmatic recess

14. 左肋膈胸膜返折线 left costodiaphragmatic line of pleural reflection
15. 右肋膈胸膜返折线 right costodiapragmatic line of pleural reflection
16. 右肋膈隐窝 right costodiaphragmatic recess
17. 膈及膈胸膜 diaphragm and diaphragmatic pleura
18. 右肺下缘 inferior margin of right lung
19. 肋胸膜 costal pleura
20. 胸骨体 body of sternum
21. 右肺 right lung
22. 胸骨柄 manubrium
23. 头臂干 brachiacephalic trunk
24. 胸膜顶 cupula of pleura
25. 迷走神经 vagus nerve

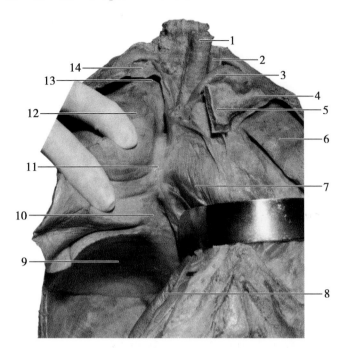

图 4-8 右肺根和肺韧带(前面观)
**Root of right lung and pulmonary
ligament(anterior view)**
1. 气管 trachea
2. 左颈总动脉 left common carotid
artery
3. 头臂干 brachiocephalic trunk
4. 第一肋 first rib
5. 胸骨柄 manubrium
6. 左肺 left lung
7. 纵隔右侧面和纵隔胸膜 right
surface of mediastinum and
mediastinal pleura
8. 膈和膈胸膜 diaphragm and
diaphragmatic pleura
9. 右肺膈面 diaphragmatic
surface of right lung
10. 肺韧带 pulmonary ligament
11. 右肺根 root of right lung
12. 右肺 right lung
13. 右肺尖 apex of right lung
14. 右胸膜顶 right cupula of pleura

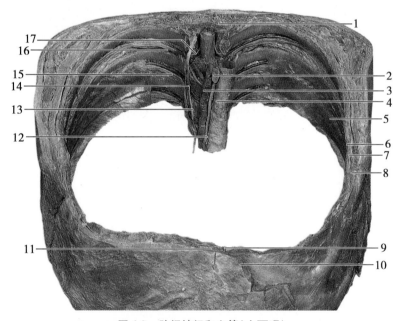

图 4-9 肋间神经和血管(上面观)
Intercostal nerves and blood vessels(superior view)

1. 竖脊肌 erector spinae
2. 后纵隔淋巴结 posterior mediasternal lymph nodes
3. 奇静脉 azygos vein
4. 胸主动脉 thoracic aorta
5. 肋 rib
6. 肋间最内肌 innermost intercostal
7. 肋间内肌 internal intercostal
8. 肋间外肌 external intercostal
9. 胸廓内动脉 internal thoracic artery
10. 腹直肌 rectus abdominis
11. 胸骨 sternum
12. 胸导管 thoracic duct
13. 内脏大神经 greater splanchnic nerve
14. 交感干 sympathetic trunk
15. 肋间后动脉 posterior intercostal artery
16. 肋间后静脉 posterior intercostal vein
17. 脊神经前支 anterior branch of spinal nerve

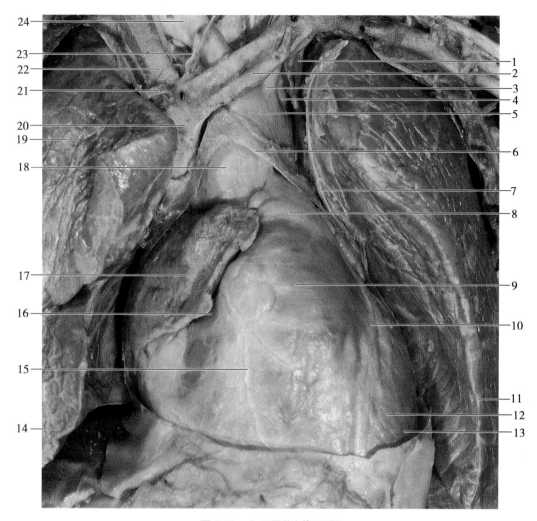

图 4-10　心于原位 (前面观)
Heart in situ (anterior view)

1. 左迷走神经 left vagus nerve
2. 左头臂静脉 left brachiocephalic vein
3. 左颈总动脉 left common carotid artery
4. 左锁骨下动脉 left subclavian artery
5. 主动脉弓 arch of aorta
6. 纤维心包 fibrous pericardium
7. 左膈神经 left phrenic nerve
8. 肺动脉干 pulmonary trunk
9. 动脉圆锥 conus arteriosus
10. 前室间沟 anterior interventricular groove
11. 左肺下叶 inferior lobe of left lung
12. 左室前壁 anterior wall of left ventricle
13. 心尖 apex of heart
14. 右肺中叶 middle lobe of right lung
15. 右室前壁 anterior wall of right ventricle
16. 右冠状沟 right coronary sulcus
17. 右心耳 right auricle
18. 升主动脉 ascending aorta
19. 右肺上叶 superior lobe of right lung
20. 上腔静脉 superior vena cava
21. 胸廓内静脉 internal thoracic vein
22. 右头臂静脉 right brachiocephalic vein
23. 甲状腺下静脉 inferior thyroid vein
24. 头臂干 brachiocephailc trunk

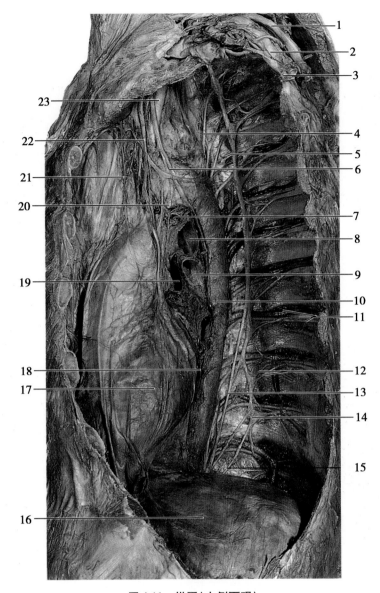

图 4-11　纵隔（左侧面观）
Mediastinum（left lateral view）

1. 臂丛外侧束 lateral cord of brachial plexus
2. 腋动脉 axillary artery
3. 臂丛内侧束 medial cord of brachial plexus
4. 肋间后动脉 posterior intercostal artery
5. 交感干 sympathetic trunk
6. 迷走神经（Ⅹ）vagus nerve（Ⅹ）
7. 淋巴结 lymph node
8. 左肺动脉 left pulmonary artery
9. 左主支气管 left principal bronchus
10. 胸主动脉 thoracic aorta
11. 肋间静脉、动脉和神经 intercostal vein,
　　 artery and nerve

12. 灰、白交通支 gray and white rami communicantes
13. 内脏大神经 greater splanchnic nerve
14. 交感神经节 sympathetic ganglion
15. 内脏小神经 lesser splanchnic nerve
16. 膈 diaphragm
17. 心包 pericardium
18. 肺韧带 pulmonary ligament
19. 左上肺静脉 left superior pulmonary vein
20. 动脉韧带 ligamentum arteriosum
21. 心包膈动脉 pericardiacophrenic artery
22. 膈神经 phrenic nerve
23. 左锁骨下动脉 left subclavian artery

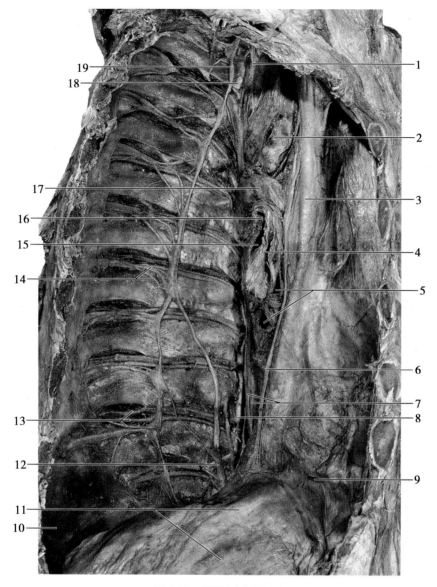

图 4-12　纵隔(右侧面观)
Mediastinum(right lateral view)

1. 右迷走神经 right vagus nerve
2. 上纵隔内淋巴结 lymph nodes in superior mediastinum
3. 上腔静脉 superior vena cava
4. 右肺动脉 right pulmonary artery
5. 右肺上、下静脉 right superior and inferior pulmonary veins
6. 右膈神经 right phrenic nerve
7. 食管及迷走神经(Ⅹ)食管丛 esophagus and esophageal plexus of vagus nerve(Ⅹ)
8. 奇静脉 azygos vein
9. 下腔静脉 inferior vena cava

10. 右肋膈隐窝 right costodiaphragmatic recess
11. 膈(覆盖膈胸膜) diaphragm(covered by pleura)
12. 内脏大神经 greater splanchnic nerve
13. 肋间神经血管 intercostal vein,artery and nerve
14. 灰、白交通支 gray and white rami communicantes
15. 中间支气管 intermediate bronchus
16. 右肺上叶支气管 superior lobar bronchus of right lung
17. 奇静脉弓 arch of azygos vein
18. 右肋间最上静脉 right highest intercostal vein
19. 胸交感干 sympathetic trunk

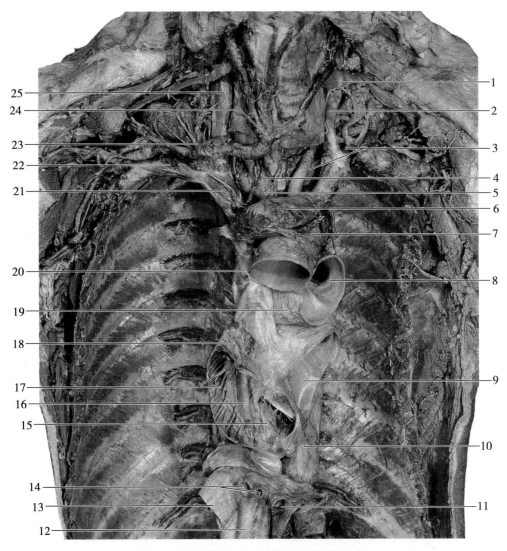

图4-13 上腔静脉、主动脉和肺动脉(前面观)
Superior vena cava, aorta and pulmonary arteries(anterior view)

1. 颈深下淋巴结 inferior cervical lymph nodes
2. 左颈内静脉 left internal jugular vein
3. 胸导管 thoracic duct
4. 右颈总动脉 right common carotid artery
5. 头臂干 brachiocephalic trunk
6. 左头臂静脉 left brachiocephalic vein
7. 主动脉弓 arch of aorta
8. 左肺动脉 left pulmonary artery
9. 左心房 left atrium
10. 食管 esophagus
11. 肝左静脉 left hepatic vein
12. 下腔静脉 inferior vena cava
13. 膈 diaphragm

14. 肝右、肝中静脉 right and middle hepatic veins
15. 右心房 right atrium
16. 界嵴 crista terminalis
17. 梳状肌 pectinate muscle
18. 右心耳 right auricle
19. 右肺动脉 right pulmonary artery
20. 上腔静脉 superior vena cava
21. 右头臂静脉 right brachiocephalic vein
22. 右锁骨下静脉 right subclavian vein
23. 右淋巴导管 right lymphatic duct
24. 甲状腺下静脉 inferior thyroid vein
25. 右颈内静脉 right internal jugular vein

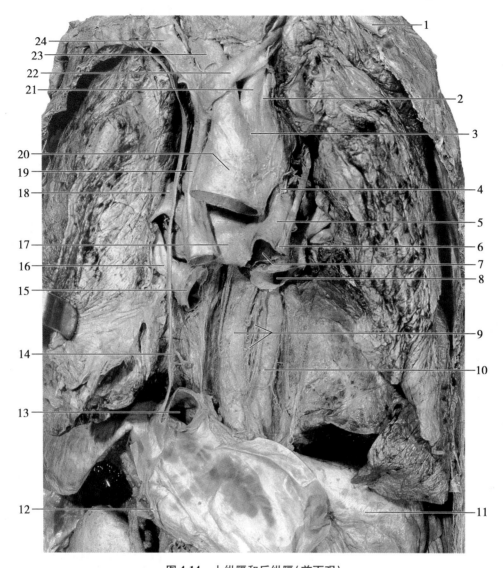

图 4-14 上纵隔和后纵隔(前面观)
Superior and posterior mediastinum(anterior view)

1. 腋动脉 axillary artery
2. 左锁骨下动脉 left subclavian artery
3. 主动脉弓 arch of aorta
4. 动脉韧带 ligamentum arteriosum
5. 左肺动脉 left pulmonary artery
6. 左迷走神经 left vagus nerve
7. 肺动脉干 pulmonary trunk
8. 左肺静脉 left pulmonary vein
9. 食管及迷走神经(Ⅹ)食管丛 esophagus and esophageal plexus of vagus nerve(Ⅹ)
10. 胸主动脉 thoracic aorta
11. 膈胸膜 diaphragmatic pleura
12. 纤维心包切断处 cut edge of fibrous pericardium

13. 下腔静脉 inferior vena cava
14. 右膈神经 right phrenic nerve
15. 右肺静脉 right pulmonary vein
16. 右下肺静脉 right inferior pulmonary vein
17. 右肺动脉 right pulmonary artery
18. 奇静脉弓 arch of azygos vein
19. 上腔静脉 superior vena cava
20. 升主动脉 ascending aorta
21. 左颈总动脉 left common carotid artery
22. 左头臂静脉 left brachiocephalic vein
23. 头臂干 brachiocephalic trunk
24. 右头臂静脉 right brachiocephalic vein

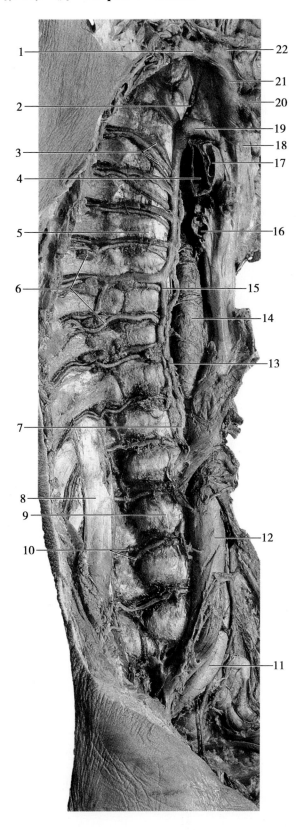

图 4-15　奇静脉和胸导管（右侧面观）
Azygos vein and thoracic duct（right lateral view）

1. 右锁骨下静脉 right subclavian vein
2. 右最上肋间静脉 right highest intercostal vein
3. 肋间神经血管 intercostal nerve and blood vessels
4. 右主支气管 right principal bronchus
5. 胸椎椎体 body of thoracic vertebra
6. 肋间后淋巴结 posterior intercostal lymph nodes
7. 乳糜池 cisterna chili
8. 腰方肌 quadratus lumborum
9. 腰椎椎体 body of lumber vertebra
10. 腰动、静脉 lumbar artery and vein
11. 右髂总动脉 right common iliac artery
12. 下腔静脉 inferior vena cava
13. 胸导管 thoracic duct
14. 食管 esophagus
15. 奇静脉 azygos vein
16. 右肺静脉 right pulmonary vein
17. 右肺动脉 right pulmonary artery
18. 上腔静脉 superior vena cava
19. 奇静脉弓 arch of azygos vein
20. 左头臂静脉 left brachiocephalic vein
21. 右头臂静脉 right brachiocephalic vein
22. 右颈内静脉 right internal jugular vein

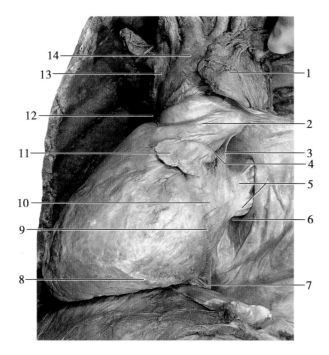

图 4-16　浆膜心包（左侧面观）
Serous pericardium（left lateral view）

1. 胸腺 thymus
2. 肺动脉干 pulmonary trunk
3. 左腔静脉襞 fold of left vena cava
4. 心包横窦 transverse pericardial sinus
5. 左上、下肺静脉 left superior and inferior pulmonary veins
6. 心包斜窦 oblique sinus of pericardium
7. 下腔静脉 inferior vena cava
8. 后室间沟 posterior interventricular groove
9. 左房斜静脉 oblique vein of left atrium
10. 左心房 left atrium
11. 左心耳 left auricle
12. 心包横窦 transverse pericardial sinus
13. 上腔静脉 superior vena cava
14. 主动脉弓 arch of aorta

图 4-17　冠状动脉和心的静脉（右前外侧面观）
Coronary arteries and cardiac veins（right anterolateral view）

1. 右心耳 right auricle
2. 窦房结支 branch to sinoatrial node
3. 右冠状动脉 right coronary artery
4. 右缘支 right marginal branch
5. 前室间支 anterior interventricular branch
6. 心前静脉 anterior cardiac vein
7. 右室前支 anterior branch of right ventricle
8. 右圆锥动脉 right conus artery
9. 升主动脉 ascending aorta

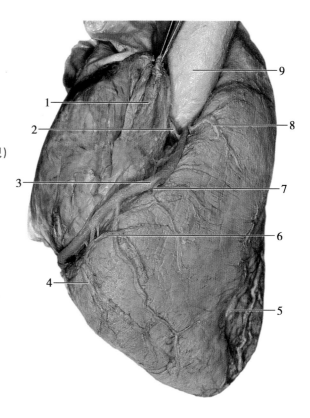

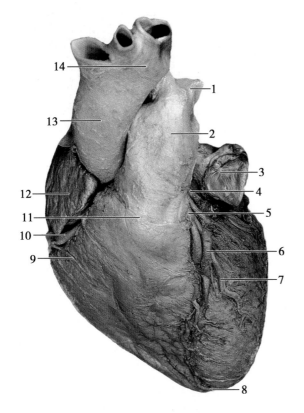

图 4-18　冠状动脉和心的静脉（左前侧面观）
Coronary arteries and cardiac veins
（left anterolateral view）

1. 左肺动脉 left pulmonary artery
2. 肺动脉干 pulmonary trunk
3. 左心耳 left auricle
4. 旋支 circumflex branch
5. 前室间支 anterior interventricular branch
6. 心大静脉 great cardiac vein
7. 左室前支 anterior branch of left ventcle
8. 心尖切迹 notch of cardiac apex
9. 右缘支 right marginal branch
10. 右冠状动脉 right coronary artery
11. 动脉圆锥 conus arteriosus
12. 右心耳 right auricle
13. 升主动脉 ascending aorta
14. 主动脉弓 arch of aorta

图 4-19　冠状动脉和心的静脉（后面观）
Coronary arteries and cardiac veins
（posterior view）

1. 左上肺静脉 left superior pulmonary vein
2. 左心房 left atrium
3. 左下肺静脉 left inferior pulmonary vein
4. 冠状窦 coronary sinus
5. 旋支 circumflex branch
6. 左缘支 left marginal branch
7. 旋支后支 posterior branch of circumflex branch
8. 左心室后壁 posterior wall of left ventricle
9. 右心室后壁 posterior wall of right ventricle
10. 后室间支 posterior interventricular branch
11. 心中静脉 middle cardiac vein
12. 右冠状动脉 right coronary artery
13. 心小静脉 small cardiac vein
14. 下腔静脉 inferior vena cava

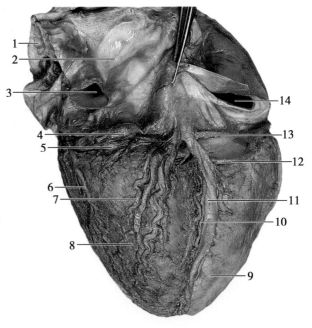

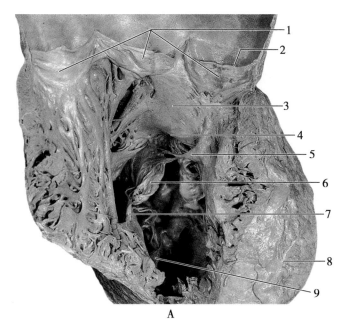

1. 肺动脉半月瓣 semilunar cusps of pulmonary valve
2. 肺动脉窦 sinus of pulmonary trunk
3. 动脉圆锥 conus arteriosus
4. 室上嵴 supraventricular crest
5. 隔侧乳头肌 septal papillary muscle
6. 三尖瓣前瓣 anterior cusp of tricuspid valve
7. 前乳头肌 anterior papillary muscle
8. 前室间支 anterior interventricular branch
9. 后乳头肌 posterior papillary muscle

A

1. 右心耳 right auricle
2. 肺动脉干 pulmonary trunk
3. 动脉圆锥 conus arteriosus
4. 室上嵴 supraventricular crest
5. 三尖瓣前瓣 anterior cusp of tricuspid valve
6. 腱索 chordae tendineae
7. 前乳头肌 anterior papillary muscle
8. 隔缘肉柱 septomarginal trabecula
9. 前室间沟 anterior interventricular groove

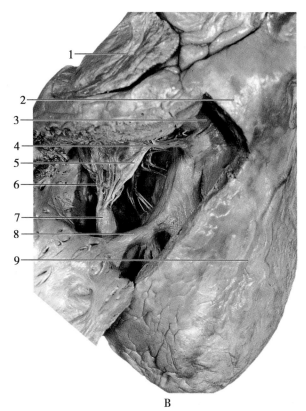

B

图 4-20　右心室（已切开）Right ventricle of heart（dissected）
A. 上面观 Superior view　B. 前面观 Anterior view

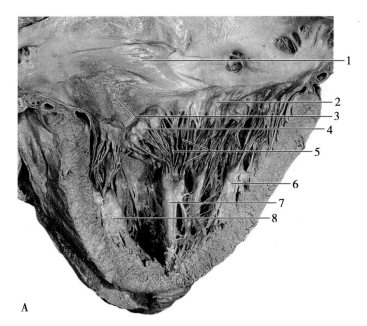

A

1. 左心房 left atrium
2. 二尖瓣后瓣 posterior cusp of mitral valve
3. 二尖瓣前瓣 anterior cusp of mitral valve
4. 纤维小结节 fibrous nodules
5. 腱索 chordae tendineae
6. 前乳头肌(已切开) anterior papillary muscle(dissected)
7. 后乳头肌 posterior papillary muscle
8. 前乳头肌(已切开) anterior papillary muscle(dissected)

1. 左冠状动脉口 orifice of left coronary artery
2. 主动脉窦 aortic sinuses
3. 右冠状动脉口 orifice of right coronary artery
4. 半月瓣小结 nodule of semilunar valve
5. 室间隔膜部 membranous part of interventricular septum
6. 二尖瓣前瓣 anterior cusp of mitral valve
7. 腱索 chordae tendineaa
8. 室间隔肌性部 muscular part of interventricular septum
9. 前乳头肌 anterior papillary muscle
10. 后乳头肌 posterior papillary muscle

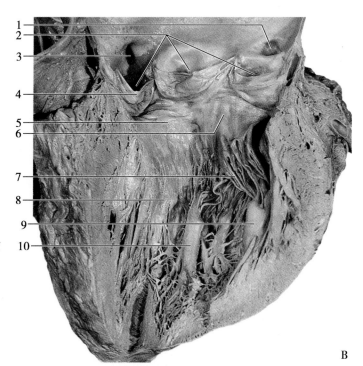

B

图 4-21 左心室(已切开) Left ventricle of heart(dissected)
A. 左侧面观 Left lateral view B. 前面观 Anterior view

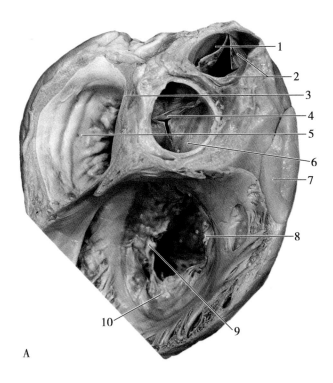

1. 肺动脉干窦 sinus of pulmonary trunk
2. 肺动脉瓣 pulmonary valve
3. 纤维环 anulus fibrous
4. 主动脉瓣 aortic valve
5. 二尖瓣后瓣 posterior cusp of mitral valve
6. 主动脉窦 aortic sinus
7. 右心耳 right auricle
8. 三尖瓣前瓣 anterior cusp of tricuspid valve
9. 三尖瓣隔侧瓣 septal cusp of tricuspid valve
10. 三尖瓣后瓣 posterior cusp of tricuspid valve

A

1. 肺动脉瓣 pulmonary valve
2. 升主动脉 ascending aorta
3. 右心耳 right auricle
4. 右纤维三角 right fibrous trigone
5. 二尖瓣前瓣 anterior cusp of mitral valve
6. 二尖瓣后瓣 posterior cusp of mitral valve
7. 三尖瓣前瓣 anterior cusp of tricuspid valve
8. 三尖瓣隔瓣 anterior cusp of tricuspid valve
9. 三尖瓣后瓣 posterior cusp of tricuspid valve

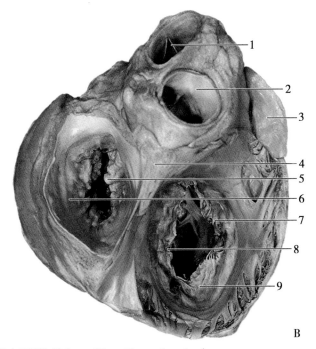

B

图 4-22 心的瓣膜（上面观）Valves of heart（superior view）
A. 主动脉瓣和肺动脉瓣 Aortic and pulmonary valves
B. 三尖瓣和二尖瓣 Tricuspid and mitral valves

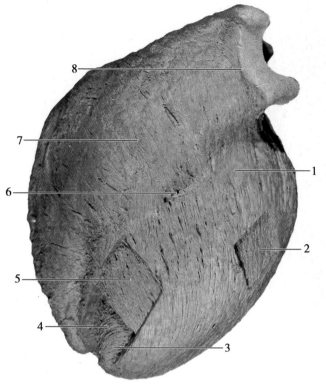

图 4-23　心肌构筑（前面观）
Myocardiac architecture
（anterior view）

1. 左心室浅层肌 superficial layer
   muscle of left ventricle
2、5. 左心室中层肌 middle layer
   muscle of left ventricle
3. 心涡 vortex of apex of heart
4. 左心室深层肌 deep layer muscle
   of left ventricle
6. 前室间沟 anterior interventricular
   groove
7. 右心室浅层肌 superficial layer
   muscle of right ventricle
8. 肺动脉干 pulmonary trunk

图 4-24　冠状动脉红色铸型
Red colored resin corrosion cast
of the coronary arteries

1. 左冠状动脉 left coronary artery
2. 左圆锥动脉 left conus artery
3. 前室间支 anterior interventricular
   branch
4. 左缘支 left marginal branch
5. 右缘支 right marginal branch
6. 右圆锥动脉 right conus artery
7. 右冠状动脉 right coronary artery

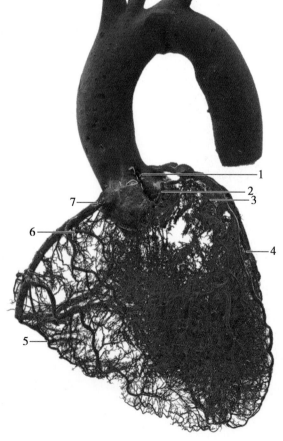

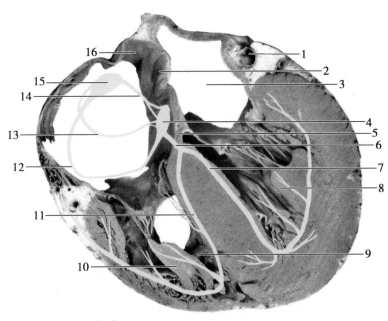

图 **4-25** 心传导系统
Cardiac conducting system

1. 左冠状动脉 left coronary artery
2. 卵圆窝 fossa ovalis
3. 左心房 left atrium
4. 房室结 atrioventricular node
5. 室间隔膜部 membranous part of interventricular septum
6. 房室束 atrioventricular bundle
7. 左束支 left bundle branch
8. 左室前乳头肌 anterior papillary muscle of the left ventricle
9. 隔缘肉柱 septomarginal trabecula
10. 右室前乳头肌 anterior papillary muscle of the right ventricle
11. 右束支 right bundle branch
12. 后结间束 posterior inter-nodal tract
13. 中结间束 middle inter-nodal tract
14. 前结间束 anterior inter-nodal tract
15. 窦房结 sinuatrial node
16. 上腔静脉口 orifice of superior vena cava

图 **4-26** 喉、气管及支气管(前面观)
Larynx,trachea and bronchi (anterior view)

1. 甲状软骨 thyroid cartilage
2. 环甲正中韧带 median cricothyroid ligament
3. 环状软骨 cricoid cartilage
4. 气管 trachea
5. 左主支气管 left principal bronchus
6. 左肺上叶支气管 left superior lobar bronchus
7. 左肺下叶支气管 left inferior lobar bronchus
8. 右肺下叶支气管 right inferior lobar bronchus
9. 右肺中叶支气管 right middle lobar bronchus
10. 右肺上叶支气管 right superior lobar bronchus
11. 右主支气管 right principal bronchus

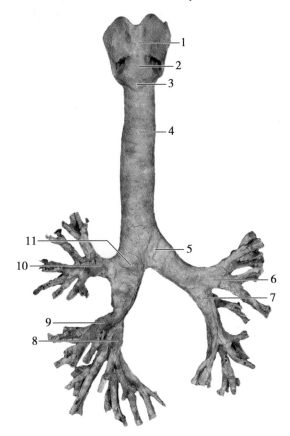

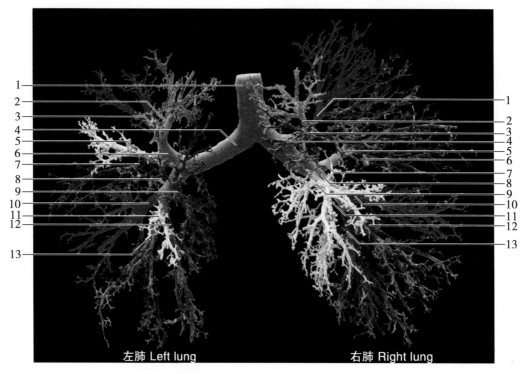

图 4-27　支气管肺段铸型（后面观）

Colored resin corrosion cast of bronchopulmonary segments（posterior view）

左肺 Left lung

1. 气管 trachea
2. 尖后段支气管 apicoposterior segmental bronchus
3. 前段支气管 anterior segmental bronchus
4. 左主支气管 left principal bronchus
5. 上舌段支气管 superior lingular segmental bronchus
6. 上叶支气管 left superior lobar bronchus
7. 下舌段支气管 inferior lingular segmental bronchus
8. 下叶支气管 left inferior lobar bronchus
9. 上段支气管 superior segmental bronchus
10. 外侧底段支气管 lateral basal segmental bronchus
11. 内侧底段支气管 medial basal segmental bronchus
12. 后底段支气管 posterior basal segmental bronchus
13. 前底段支气管 anterior basal segmental bronchus

右肺 Right lung

1. 前段支气管 anterior segmental bronchus
2. 尖段支气管 apical segmental bronchus
3. 后段支气管 posterior segmental bronchus
4. 上叶支气管 right superior lobar bronchus
5. 内侧段支气管 medial segmental bronchus
6. 外侧段支气管 lateral segmental bronchus
7. 中叶支气管 right middle lobar bronchus
8. 下叶支气管 right inferior lobar bronchus
9. 上段支气管 superior segmental bronchus
10. 外侧底段支气管 lateral basal segmental bronchus
11. 内侧底段支气管 medial basal segmental bronchus
12. 前底段支气管 anterior basal segmental bronchus
13. 后底段支气管 posterior basal segmental bronchus

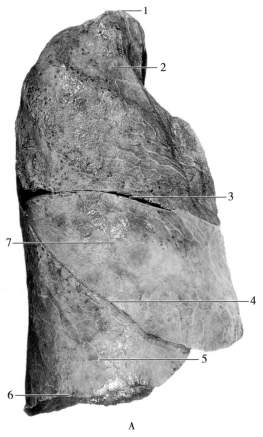

A

1. 右肺尖 apex of right lung
2. 上叶 upper lobe of right lung
3. 水平裂 horizontal fissure
4. 斜裂 oblique fissure
5. 下叶 lower lobe of right lung
6. 下缘 inferior margin
7. 中叶 middle lobe of right lung
8. 第一肋压迹 impression for first rib
9. 上腔静脉压迹 impression for
   superior vena cava
10. 右肺动脉上支 superior branch of right
    pulmonary artery
11. 上肺静脉 superior pulmonary vein
12. 心压迹 cardiac impression
13. 膈面 diaphragmatic surface

14. 肺韧带 pulmonary ligament
15. 下肺静脉 inferior pulmonary vein
16. 右肺动脉下支 inferior branch of
    right pulmonary artery
17. 中间支气管 intermediate bronchus
18. 上叶支气管 superior lobar bronchus
19. 奇静脉压迹 impression for azygos
    vein

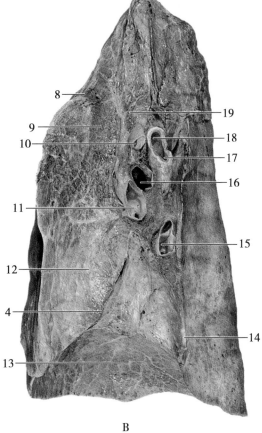

B

图 4-28　右肺 Right lung
　A. 肋面 Costal surface
　B. 纵隔面 Mediastinal surface

1. 左肺尖 apex of left lung
2. 上叶 upper lobe of left lung
3. 斜裂 oblique fissure
4. 下缘 inferior margin
5. 下叶 lower lobe of left lung

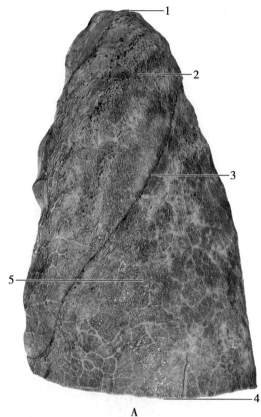

A

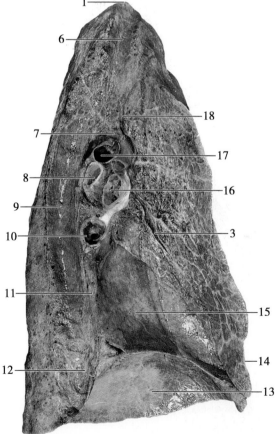

6. 食管压迹 impression for esophagus
7. 主动脉弓压迹 impression for arch of aorta
8. 左主支气管 left principal bronchus
9. 降主动脉压迹 impression for descending aorta
10. 下肺静脉 inferior pulmonary vein
11. 肺韧带 pulmonary ligament
12. 食管压迹 impression for esophagus
13. 膈面 diaphragmatic surface
14. 心切迹 cardiac notch
15. 心压迹 cardiac impression
16. 上肺静脉 superior pulmonary vein
17. 肺动脉 left pulmonary artery
18. 左锁骨下动脉压迹 impression for left subclavian artery

图 4-29　左肺 Left lung
A. 肋面 Costal surface　B. 纵隔面 Mediastinal surface

B

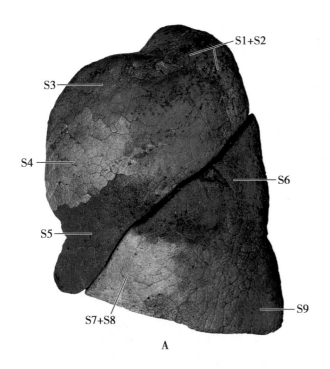

S1+S2 尖后段 apicoposterior segment
S3 前段 anterior segment
S4 上舌段 superior lingular segment
S5 下舌段 inferior lingular segment
S6 上段 superior segment
S7+S8 内侧底段（又称心底段）medial
　　　basal segment（cardiac basal
　　　segmental+前底段 anterior
　　　basal segment）
S9 外侧底段 lateral basal segmental
S10 后底段 posterior basal segmental

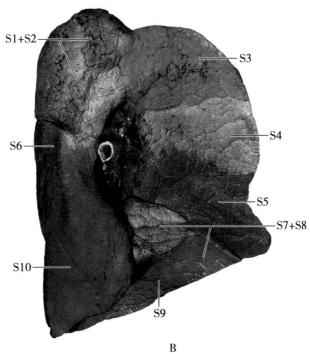

图 4-30 染料灌注示意左肺支气管肺段
Colored territories for bronchopulmonary segments of left lung
A. 肋面 Costal surface B. 纵隔面 Mediastinal surface

95

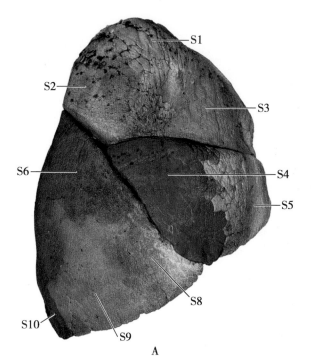

S1 尖段 apical segment
S2 后段 posterior segment
S3 前段 anterior segment
S4 外侧段 lateral segment
S5 内侧段 medial segmental
S6 上段 superior segment
S7 内侧底段(心底段)medial segment
  (cardiac basal segment)
S8 前底段 anterior basal segment
S9 外侧底段 lateral basal segment
S10 后底段支气管 posterior basal segment

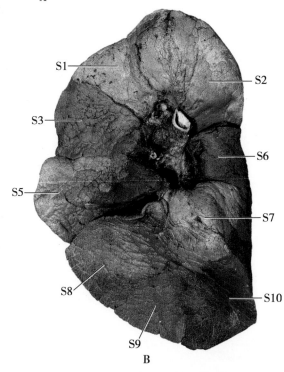

图 4-31 染料灌注示意右肺支气管肺段
Colored territories for bronchopulmonary segments of right lung
A. 肋面 Costal surface   B. 纵隔面 Mediastinal surface

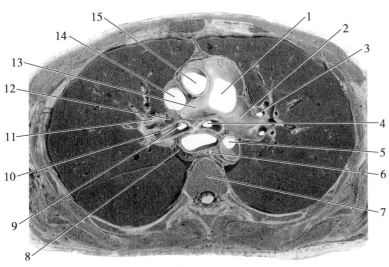

1. 肺动脉干 pulmonary trunk
2. 左肺动脉 left pulmonary artery
3. 左上叶支气管 left superior lobar bronchus
4. 左主支气管 left principal bronchus
5. 胸主动脉 thoracic aorta
6. 胸导管 thoracic duct
7. 胸椎椎体 body of thoracic vertebra
8. 奇静脉 azygos vein
9. 右主支气管 right principal bronchus
10. 右肺上叶支气管 right superior lobar bronchus
11. 右上肺静脉 right superior pulmonary vein
12. 右肺动脉上支 superior branch of right pulmonary artery
13. 右肺动脉 right pulmonary artery
14. 上腔静脉 superior vena cava
15. 升主动脉 ascending aorta

图 4-32　经肺动脉分叉胸部横断面（下面观）
Transverse section through thorax at level of bifurcation of pulmonary trunk（inferior view）

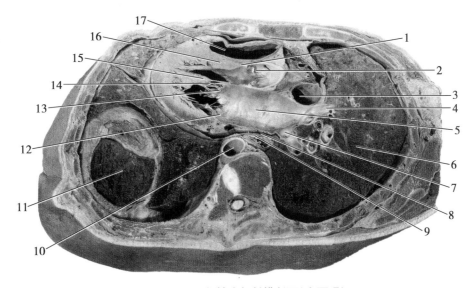

图 4-33　经心长轴胸部斜横断面（上面观）
Oblique transverse section through thorax at long axis of heart（superior view）

1. 室间隔膜部 membranous part of interventricular septum
2. 主动脉口右窦、右冠状动脉口 right sinus of aortic orifice and orifice of right coronary artery
3. 上腔静脉 superior vena cava
4. 右上肺静脉 right superior pulmonary vein
5. 左心房 left atrium
6. 右肺上叶 superior lobe of right lung
7. 右下肺静脉 right inferior pulmonary vein
8. 心包斜窦 oblique sinus of pericardium
9. 食管 esophagus
10. 胸主动脉 thoracic aorta
11. 脾 spleen
12. 二尖瓣后瓣 posterior cusp of mitral valve
13. 二尖瓣前瓣 anterior cusp of mitral valve
14. 腱索 chordae tendineae
15. 前乳头肌 anterior papillary muscle
16. 室间隔间性部 muscular part of interventricular septum
17. 右心室 right ventricle

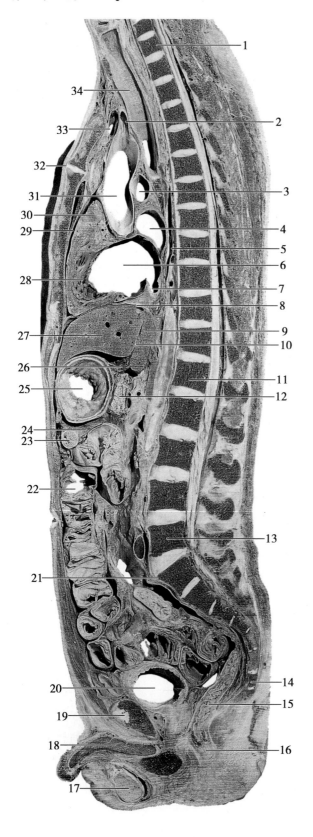

图 **4-34** 躯干正中矢状断面（左侧面观）
Median sagittal section of trunk
(left lateral view)

1. 第一胸椎椎体 body of first thoracic vertebra
2. 头臂干 brachiocephalic trunk
3. 右肺动脉 right pulmonary artery
4. 左心房 left atrium
5. 食管 esophagus
6. 右心房 right atrium
7. 下腔静脉 inferior vena cava
8. 冠状韧带上层 superior layer of coronary
9. 肝尾状叶 caudate lobe of liver
10. 静脉韧带裂及肝胃韧带 fissure for ligmentum venosum and hepatogastric ligament
11. 第一腰椎椎体 body of first lumber vertebra
12. 胰 pancreas
13. 第五腰椎椎体 body of fifth lumber vertebra
14. 尾骨 coccyx
15. 直肠 rectum
16. 肛门 anus
17. 睾丸 testis
18. 阴茎 penis
19. 耻骨联合 pubic symphysis
20. 膀胱 urinary bladder
21. 骶岬 promontory of sacrum
22. 小肠 jejunum
23. 横结肠 transverse colon
24. 横结肠系膜 transverse mesocolon
25. 胃 stomach
26. 肝胃韧带 hepatogastric ligament
27. 肝 liver
28. 右心室 right ventricle
29. 心包腔 serous pericardial cavity
30. 右心耳 right auriche
31. 升主动脉 ascending aorta
32. 胸骨角 sternal angle
33. 左头臂静脉 left brachiocephalic vein
34. 气管 trachea

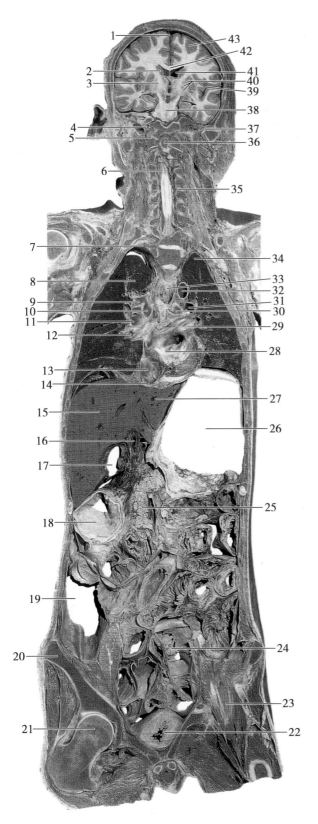

图 4-35 经齿突头、颈和躯干冠状断面 (前面观)
Coronary section through head, neck and trunk at level of dens of axis (anterior view)

1. 大脑镰 falx cerebri
2. 尾状核 caudate nucleus
3. 内囊 internal capsule
4. 颈内动脉 internal carotid artery
5. 寰枕关节 atlantooccipital joint
6. 脊髓 spinal cord
7. 胸膜顶 (颈胸膜) cupula (cervical pleura)
8. 右肺上叶 superior lobe of right lung
9. 右肺下叶支气管 right inferior lobar bronchus
10. 右中间支气管 right intermediate bronchus
11. 右肺动脉 right pulmonary artery
12. 右肺下叶支气管 right inferior lobar bronchus
13. 右心房 right atrium
14. 下腔静脉 inferior vena cava
15. 肝右叶 right lobe of liver
16. 肝门静脉 hepatic portal vein
17. 胆囊 gallbladder
18. 横结肠右曲 right colic flexure
19. 升结肠 ascending colon
20. 髂骨 ilium
21. 股骨头 head of femur
22. 膀胱 urinary bladder
23. 髂腰肌 iliopsoas
24. 空肠 jejunum
25. 胰体 body of pancreas
26. 胃 stomach
27. 肝左叶 left lobe of liver
28. 左心房 left atrium
29. 左肺静脉 left pulmonary vein
30. 左主支气管 left principal bronchus
31. 左肺动脉 left pulmonary artery
32. 主动脉弓 arch of aorta
33. 食管 esophagus
34. 左肺尖 apex of left lung
35. 颈椎椎间关节 cervical intervertebral joint
36. 枢椎齿突 dens of axis
37. 颞下颌关节盘 articular disc of temporomandibular joint
38. 脑桥 pons
39. 大脑半球外侧沟 lateral sulcus of cerebral hemisphere
40. 豆状核 lentiform nucleus
41. 侧脑室 lateral ventricle
42. 胼胝体 corpus callosum
43. 顶叶 parietal lobe

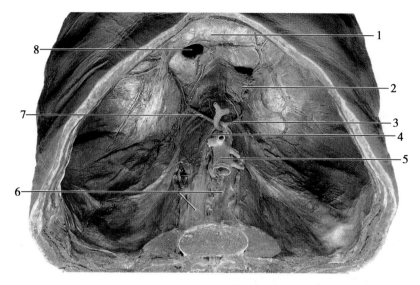

图 4-36 膈（下面观）
Diaphragm（inferior view）

1. 膈中心腱 central tendon of diaphragm
2. 食管腹段 abdominal part of esophagus
3. 左膈下动脉 left inferior phrenic artery
4. 主动脉裂孔 aortic hiatus

5. 腹主动脉 abdominal aorta
6. 左、右膈脚 left and right crura of diaphragm
7. 右膈下动脉 right inferior phrenic artery
8. 腔静脉孔 caval opening

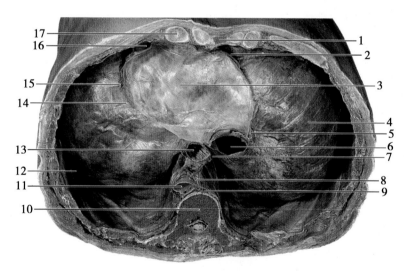

图 4-37 膈（上面观）
Diaphragm（superior view）

1. 胸骨 sternum
2. 右肋膈隐窝 right costodiaphragmatic recess
3. 膈中心腱（被纤维心包覆盖）central tendon of diaphragm（covered by pericardium）
4. 膈肌性部 muscular part of diaphragm
5. 右膈神经和心包膈动脉、静脉 right phrenic nerve and pericardiophrenic artery and vein
6. 下腔静脉 inferior vena cava
7. 食管隐窝 esophageal recess
8. 胸导管 thoracic duct

9. 奇静脉 azygos vein
10. 胸椎椎体 body of thoracic vertebra
11. 胸主动脉 thoracic aorta
12. 左肋膈隐窝 left costodiaphragmatic recess
13. 食管 esophagus
14. 纤维心包切断处 cut edge of fibrous pericardium
15. 左膈神经和心包膈动脉、静脉 left phrenic nerve and pericardiophrenic artery and vein
16. 左肋纵隔窦 left costomediastinal recess
17. 肋软骨 costal cartilage

100

第 5 章　腹

Chapter 5　Abdomen

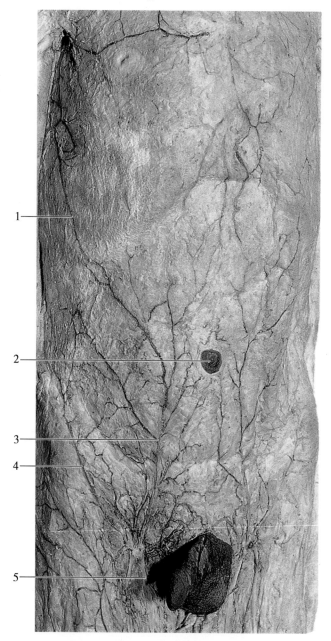

图 5-1 腹前外侧壁的浅静脉（前面观）
Superficial veins on anterolateral wall of
abdomen（anterior view）

1. 胸腹壁静脉 thoracoepigastirc vein
2. 脐 umbilicus
3. 腹壁浅静脉 superficial epigastric vein
4. 旋髂浅静脉 superficial circumflex iliac vein
5. 大隐静脉 great saphenous vein

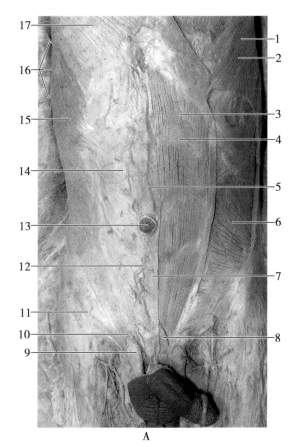

A

1. 前锯肌 serratus anterior
2、15. 腹外斜肌 obliquus externus abdominis
3. 腹直肌 rectus abdominis
4. 腱划 tendinous intersection
5、7. 腹白线 linea alba
6. 腹内斜肌 obliquus internus abdominis
8. 锥状肌 pyramidalis
9. 精索 spermatic cord
10. 腹股沟管浅环 superficial inguinal ring
11. 腹股沟韧带 inguinal ligament
12. 第十一胸脊神经前皮支 anterior cutaneous branch of eleventh thoracic spinal nerve
13. 脐 umbilicus
14. 腹直肌鞘前层 anterior layer of sheath of rectus abdominis
16. 胸脊神经外侧皮支 lateral cutaneous branches of thoracic spinal nerves
17. 胸大肌 pectoralis major

1. 腹壁上动脉、静脉 superior epigastric artery and vein
2. 腹外斜肌 obliquus externus abdominis
3. 腹直肌鞘后层 posterior layer of sheath of rectus abdominis
4. 左第十胸脊神经前支 anterior branch of left tenth thoracic spinal nerve
5. 腹壁下动脉、静脉 inferior epigastric artery and vein
6. 腹股沟管浅环 superficial inguinal ring
7. 精索 spermatic cord
8. 髂腹股沟神经 ilioinguinal nerve
9. 髂腹下神经 iliohypogastric nerve
10. 腹直肌鞘前层 anterior layer of sheath of rectus abdominis
11. 腹横肌 transversus abdominis
12. 右第十胸脊神经前支 anterior branch of right tenth thoracic spinal nerve
13. 腹内斜肌 obliquus internus abdominis

图 5-2　腹前外侧壁的肌和腱膜（前面观）
Muscles and aponeurosis of anterolateral abdominal wall（anterior view）
A. 右腹外斜肌、左腹直肌和左腹内斜肌 Right obliquus externus abdorminis, left rectus abdominis and left obliquus internus abdominis　B. 右腹横肌和左腹直肌鞘后层 Right transversus abdominis and posterior layer of sheath of rectus abdominis

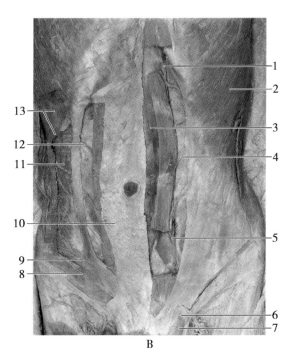

B

103

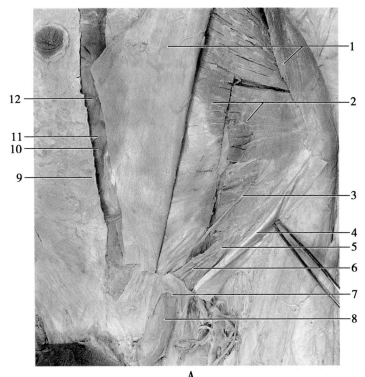

1. 腹外斜肌 obliquus externus abdominis
2、15. 腹内斜肌 obliquus internus abdominis
3. 髂腹下神经 iliohypogastric nerve
4. 腹股沟韧带 inguinal ligament
5、8、19. 精索 spermatic cord
6. 髂腹股沟神经 ilioinguinal nerve
7、20. 腹股沟管浅环 superficial inguinal ring
9. 腹直肌鞘前层 anterior layer of sheath of rectus abdominis
10、14、24. 腹横筋膜 transversalis fascia

11、25. 弓状线 arcuate line
12、26. 腹直肌鞘后层 posterior layer of sheath of rectus abdominis
13、16. 腹横肌 transversus abdominis
17. 腹股沟管深环 deep inguinal ring
18. 凹间韧带 interfoveolar ligament
21. 腹股沟镰（联合腱）inguinal falx（conjoint tendon）
22. 锥状肌 pyramidalis
23. 腹直肌 rectus abdominis

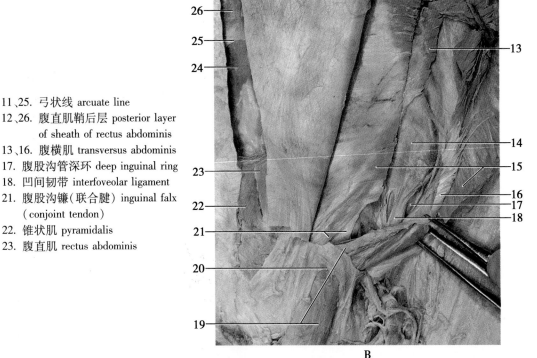

图 5-3 左侧腹股沟管（前面观）
Left inguinal canal（anterior view）
A. 浅环 Superficial ring B. 深环 Deep ring

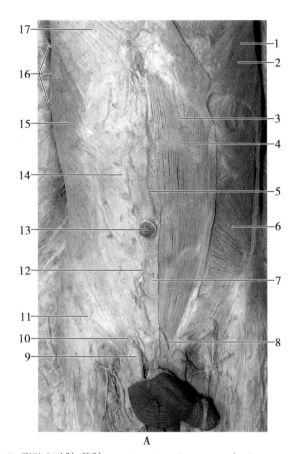

A

1. 前锯肌 serratus anterior
2、15. 腹外斜肌 obliquus externus abdominis
3. 腹直肌 rectus abdominis
4. 腱划 tendinous intersection
5、7. 腹白线 linea alba
6. 腹内斜肌 obliquus internus abdominis
8. 锥状肌 pyramidalis
9. 精索 spermatic cord
10. 腹股沟管浅环 superficial inguinal ring
11. 腹股沟韧带 inguinal ligament
12. 第十一胸脊神经前皮支 anterior cutaneous branch of eleventh thoracic spinal nerve
13. 脐 umbilicus
14. 腹直肌鞘前层 anterior layer of sheath of rectus abdominis
16. 胸脊神经外侧皮支 lateral cutaneous branches of thoracic spinal nerves
17. 胸大肌 pectoralis major

1. 腹壁上动脉、静脉 superior epigastric artery and vein
2. 腹外斜肌 obliquus externus abdominis
3. 腹直肌鞘后层 posterior layer of sheath of rectus abdominis
4. 左第十胸脊神经前支 anterior branch of left tenth thoracic spinal nerve
5. 腹壁下动脉、静脉 inferior epigastric artery and vein
6. 腹股沟管浅环 superficial inguinal ring
7. 精索 spermatic cord
8. 髂腹股沟神经 ilioinguinal nerve
9. 髂腹下神经 iliohypogastric nerve
10. 腹直肌鞘前层 anterior layer of sheath of rectus abdominis
11. 腹横肌 transversus abdominis
12. 右第十胸脊神经前支 anterior branch of right tenth thoracic spinal nerve
13. 腹内斜肌 obliquus internus abdominis

图 5-2　腹前外侧壁的肌和腱膜（前面观）
Muscles and aponeurosis of anterolateral abdominal wall（anterior view）
A. 右腹外斜肌、左腹直肌和右腹内斜肌 Right obliquus externus abdorminis，left rectus abdominis and left obliquus internus abdominis　B. 右腹横肌和左腹直肌鞘后层 Right transversus abdominis and posterior layer of sheath of rectus abdominis

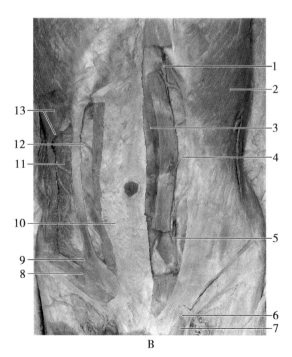

B

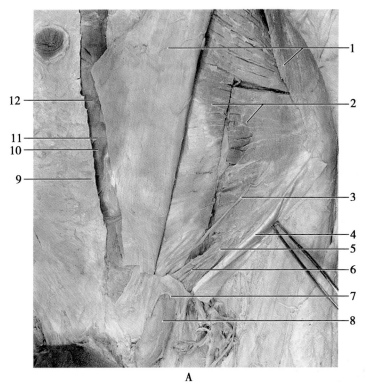

A

1. 腹外斜肌 obliquus externus abdominis
2、15. 腹内斜肌 obliquus internus abdominis
3. 髂腹下神经 iliohypogastric nerve
4. 腹股沟韧带 inguinal ligament
5、8、19. 精索 spermatic cord
6. 髂腹股沟神经 ilioinguinal nerve
7、20. 腹股沟管浅环 superficial inguinal ring
9. 腹直肌鞘前层 anterior layer of sheath of rectus abdominis
10、14、24. 腹横筋膜 transversalis fascia

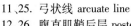

11、25. 弓状线 arcuate line
12、26. 腹直肌鞘后层 posterior layer of sheath of rectus abdominis
13、16. 腹横肌 transversus abdominis
17. 腹股沟管深环 deep inguinal ring
18. 凹间韧带 interfoveolar ligament
21. 腹股沟镰（联合腱）inguinal falx（conjoint tendon）
22. 锥状肌 pyramidalis
23. 腹直肌 rectus abdominis

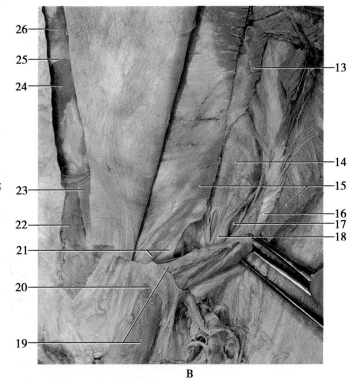

B

图 5-3 左侧腹股沟管（前面观）
Left inguinal canal（anterior view）
A. 浅环 Superficial ring B. 深环 Deep ring

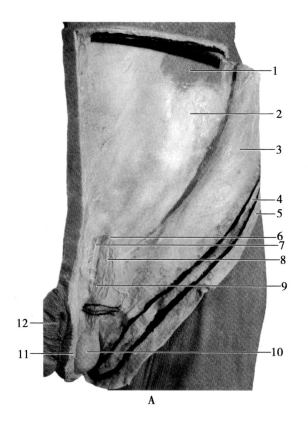

A

1. 腹外斜肌 obliquus externus abdominis
2. 腹外斜肌腱膜 aponeurosis of obliquus externus abdominis
3. 浅筋膜膜性层（斯卡帕筋膜）membranous layer of superficial fascia（Scarpa fascia）
4. 浅筋膜脂性层（坎珀尔筋膜）fatty layer of superficial fascia（Camper fascia）
5. 皮肤 skin
6. 腹股沟管浅环 superficial inguinal ring
7. 髂腹股沟神经 ilioinguinal nerve
8. 生殖股神经生殖支 genital branch of genitofemoral nerve

9. 精索 spermatic cord
10. 睾丸 testis
11. 阴囊 scrotum
12. 阴茎 penis
13. 腹股沟韧带 inguinal ligament
14. 腹股沟镰（联合腱）inguinal falx（conjoint tendon）
15. 髂腹下神经 iliohypogastric nerve
16. 腹直肌鞘前层 anterior layer of sheath of rectus abdominis
17. 腹内斜肌 obliquus internus abdominis

图 5-4 左侧腹前外壁与精索的关系（Ⅰ）（前面观）Relationships of left half of anterolateral abdominal wall to spermatic cord（Ⅰ）（anterior view）
A. 剖露腹外斜肌腱膜 aponeurosis of obliquus externus abdominis has been seen. B. 剖露腹内斜肌 obliquus internus abdominis has been seen

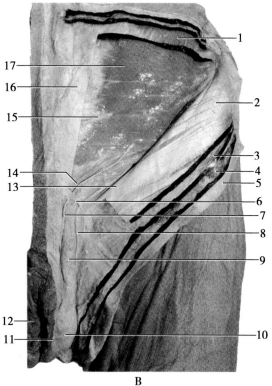

B

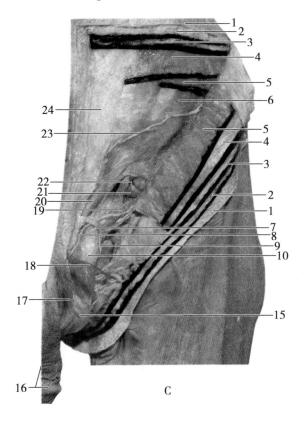

C

1. 皮肤 skin
2. 浅筋膜脂性层（坎珀尔筋膜）fatty layer of superficial fascia（Camper fascia）
3. 浅筋膜膜性层（斯卡帕筋膜）membranous layer of superficial fascia（Scarpa fascia）
4. 腹外斜肌 obliquus externus abdominis
5. 腹内斜肌 obliquus internus abdominis
6. 腹横肌 transversus abdominis
7. 腹股沟管浅环 superficial inguinal ring
8. 髂腹股沟神经 ilioinguinal nerve
9. 生殖股神经生殖支 genital branch of genitofemoral nerve
10. 精索 spermatic cord
11. 睾丸静脉 testicular vein
12. 睾丸动脉 testicular artery
13. 输精管 vas deferens
14. 附睾头 head of epididymis

15. 睾丸 testis
16. 阴茎 penis
17. 阴囊 scrotum
18. 阴部外动脉 external pudendal artery
19. 提睾肌 cremaster
20. 腹股沟镰（联合腱）inguinal falx（conjoint tendon）
21. 腹壁下动脉 inferior epigastric artery
22. 腹股沟管深环 deep inguinal ring
23. 髂腹下神经 iliohypogastric nerve
24. 腹直肌鞘前层 anterior layer of sheath of rectus abdominis
25. 腹股沟韧带 inguinal ligament
26. 锥状肌 pyramidalis
27. 腹直肌 rectus abdominis
28. 旋髂深动脉、静脉 deep circumflex iliac artery and vein
29. 半月线 linea semilunaris

图 5-4 左侧腹前外壁与精索的关系（Ⅱ）（前面观）Relationships of left half of anterolateral abdominal wall to spermatic cord（Ⅱ）（anterior view）
C. 剖露腹横肌 Transversus abdominis has been reflected D. 剖露精索被膜 Testis has been seen

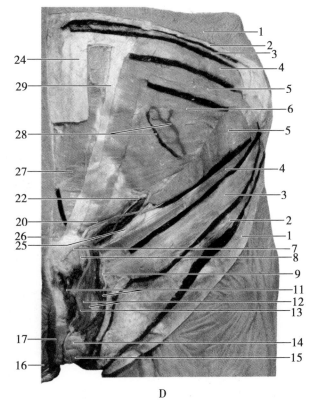

D

106

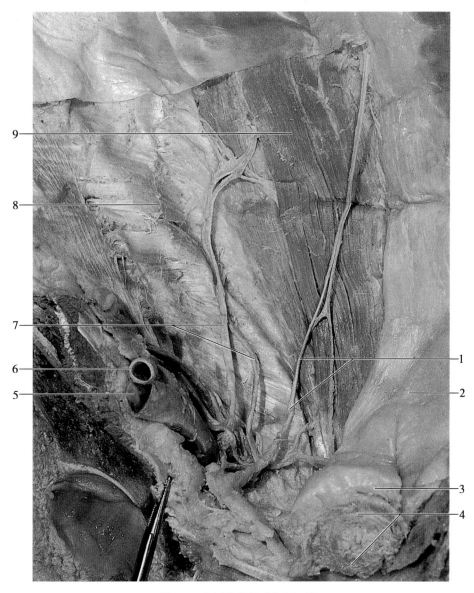

图 5-5　左侧腹前外壁(后面观)
Left half of anterolateral abdominal wall(posterior view)

1. 脐内侧韧带 medial umbilical ligament
2. 腹膜 peritoneum
3. 腹膜外筋膜 extraperitoneal fascia
4. 膀胱 urinary bladder
5. 髂外静脉 external iliac vein
6. 髂外动脉 external iliac artery
7. 腹壁下动脉、静脉 inferior epigastric artery and vein
8. 腹横肌 transversus abdominis
9. 腹直肌 rectus abdominis

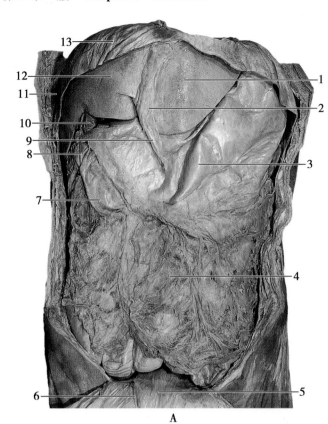

1. 肝左叶 left lobe of liver
2. 镰状韧带 falciform ligament
3. 胃 stomach
4. 大网膜 greater omentum
5. 脐正中襞 median umbilical fold
6. 左脐内侧襞 left medial umbilical fold
7. 横结肠 transverse colon
8. 结肠右曲 right colic flexure
9. 肝圆韧带 round ligament of liver
10. 胆囊 gallbladder
11. 肋膈隐窝 costodiaphragmatic recess
12. 肝右叶 right lobe of liver
13. 膈 diaphragm

A

1. 大网膜 greater omentum
2. 横结肠 transverse colon
3. 空肠 jejunum
4. 降结肠 descending colon
5. 乙状结肠 sigmoid colon
6. 回肠 ileum
7. 结肠右曲 right colic flexure

图 5-6　腹腔内器官（前面观）
The organs in abdominal cavity
（anterior view）
A. 腹前外侧壁已被下翻 Anterolateral abdominal wall has been reflected downward　B. 大网膜向上翻起 Great omentum has been reflected upward

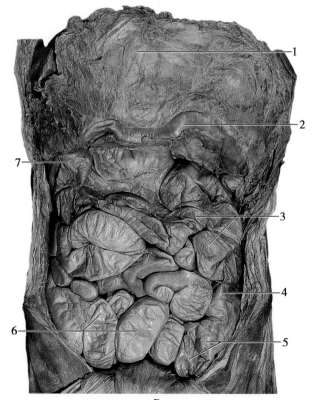

B

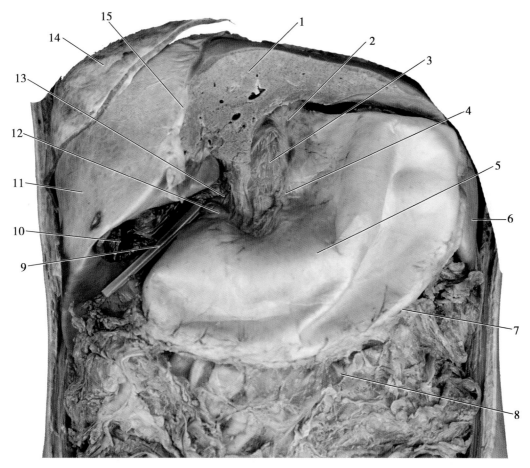

图 5-7　网膜囊前壁(前面观)
Anterior wall of omenta bursa(anterior view)

1. 肝左叶(部分切除) left lobe of liver
   (some part has been removed)
2. 食管 esophagus
3. 小网膜的肝胃韧带 hepatogastric
   ligament of lesser omentum
4. 胃小弯 lesser curvature of stomach
5. 胃 stomach
6. 脾 spleen
7. 胃大弯 greater curvature of stomach
8. 大网膜 greater omentum

9. 绿色导管(经网膜孔进网膜囊) green catheter
   (enters omenta bursa through omental foramen)
10. 胆囊 gallbladder
11. 肝右叶 right lobe of liver
12. 十二指肠上部 superior part of duodenum
13. 小网膜的肝十二指肠韧带 hepatoduodenal
    ligament of lesser omentum
14. 膈 diaphragm
15. 镰状韧带 falciform ligament

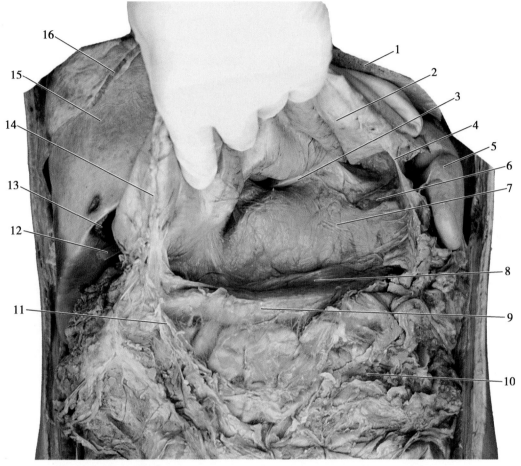

图 5-8　网膜囊后壁（沿胃大弯切开大网膜并向上翻起胃，前面观）
Posterior wall of omenta bursa（greater omentum has been dissected and stomach has been raised upward，anterior view）

1. 膈 diaphragm
2. 胃 stomach
3. 绿色导管左侧端（位于网膜囊内）left end of green catheter（lies in omenta bursa）
4. 胃脾韧带 gastrosplenic ligament
5. 脾 spleen
6. 脾静脉 splenic vein
7. 胰体 body of pancreas
8. 横结肠系膜 transverse mesocolon
9. 横结肠 transverse colon
10. 大网膜 greater omentum

11. 大网膜切断缘 cut edge of greater omentum
12. 绿色导管右侧端（位于网膜孔右侧）right end of green catheters（lies on right side of omental foramen）
13. 胆囊 gallbladder
14. 胃大弯（与大网膜的附着已被切断）greater curvature of stomach（its attachment with greater omentum has been cut）
15. 肝右叶 right lobe of liver
16. 膈 diaphragm

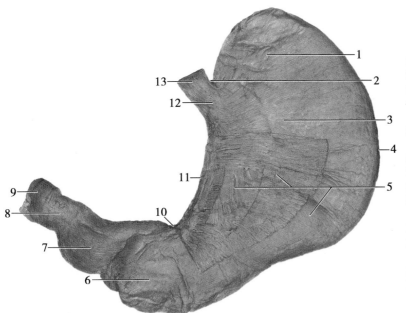

1. 胃底 fundus of stomach
2. 贲门切迹 cardiac notch
3. 胃体 body of stomach
4. 胃大弯 greater curvature of stomach
5. 胃肌层 muscle layer of stomach
6. 幽门窦 pyloric antrum
7. 幽门管 pyloric canal
8. 幽门 pylorus
9. 十二指肠上部 superior part of duodenum
10. 角切迹 angular notch
11. 胃小弯 lesser curvature of stomach
12. 贲门部 cardiac part
13. 食管腹部 abdominal part of esophagus

图 5-9　胃的外形与分部（前面观）
External appearance and subdivision of stomach（anterior view）

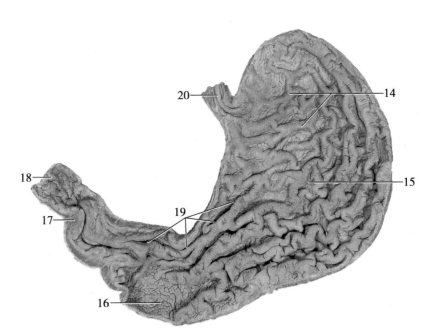

图 5-10　胃黏膜（胃前壁已切除，前面观）
Internal appearance of stomach（anterior wall of stomach has been removed，anterior view）

14. 胃黏膜皱襞 gastric folds
15、16. 胃小凹 gastric pit
17. 幽门括约肌 pyloric sphincter
18. 十二指肠皱襞 folds of duodenum
19. 胃路 gastric canal
20. 食管纵皱襞 longitudinal folds of esophagus

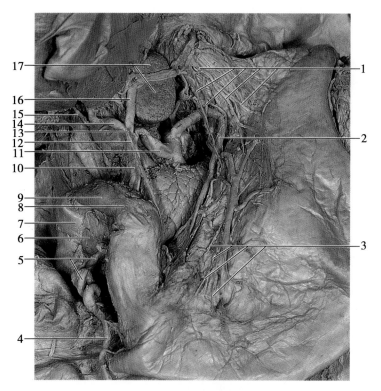

图 5-11 胃小弯的神经血管（前面观）
Nerves and blood vessels along lesser curvature of stomach（anterior view）

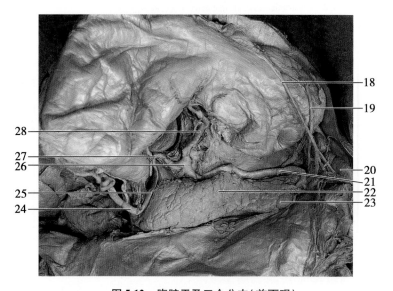

图 5-12 腹腔干及三个分支（前面观）
Celiac trunk and its three branches（anterior view）

1. 迷走神经前干分支 branches of anterior vagal trunk
2、28. 胃左动脉 left gastric artery
3. 胃前大神经 greater anterior gastric nerves
4、24. 胃网膜右动脉 right gastroepiploic artery
5、10、25. 胃十二指肠动脉 gastroduodenal artery
6. 胰头 head of pancreas
7. 十二指肠降部 descending part of duodenum
8. 幽门 pylorus
9. 十二指肠上部 superior part of duodenum
11、27. 肝总动脉 common hepatic artery
12. 胃右动脉 right gastric artery
13. 肝固有动脉 proper hepatic artery
14. 肝右动脉 right hepatic artery
15. 胆囊动脉 cystic artery
16. 肝左动脉 left hepatic artery
17. 肝尾状叶 caudate lobe of liver
18. 胃网膜左动脉 left gastroepiploic artery
19. 胃短动脉 short gastric artery
20. 脾 spleen
21. 脾动脉 splenic artery
22. 胰体 body of pancreas
23. 胰尾 tail of pancreas
26. 腹腔干 celiac trunk

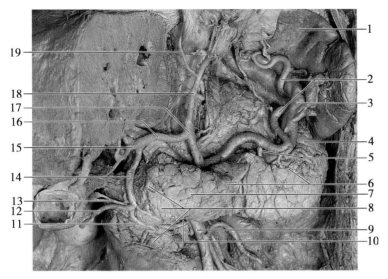

图 5-13　腹腔干与胰（前面观）
Celiac trunk and pancreas（anterior view）

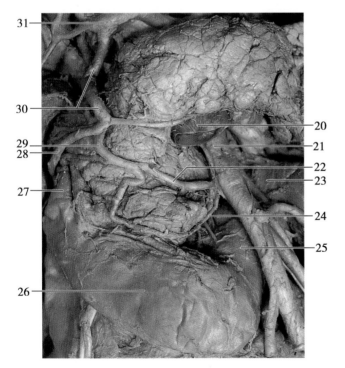

图 5-14　肠系膜上动脉与胰头（前面观）
Superior mesenteric artery and head of pancreas（anterior view）

1. 脾 spleen
2. 脾动脉 splenic artery
3. 脾静脉 splenic vein
4. 胰尾 tail of pancreas
5. 脾动脉胰支 pancreatic branches of splenic artery
6. 胰体 body of pancreas
7. 胰颈 neck of pancreas
8. 胰头 head of pancreas
9、21. 肠系膜上动脉 superior mesenteric artery
10、20. 肠系膜上静脉 superior mesenteric vein
11、29. 胰十二指肠前上动脉 anterior superior pancreaticoduodenal artery
12、28. 胃网膜右动脉 right gastroepiploic artery
13. 胰十二指肠后上动脉 posterior superior pancreaticoduodenal artery
14、30. 胃十二指肠动脉 gastroduodenal artery
15、31. 肝固有动脉 proper hepatic artery
16. 肝总动脉 common hepatic artery
17. 腹腔干 celiac trunk
18. 胃左动脉 left gastric artery
19. 胃左动脉食管支 esophageal branch of left gastric artery
22. 胰十二指肠前下动脉 anterior inferior pancreaticoduodenal artery
23. 十二指肠空肠曲 duodenojejunal flexure
24. 胰十二指肠后下动脉 posterior inferior pancreaticoduodenal artery
25. 十二指肠升部 ascending part of duodenum
26. 十二指肠水平部 horizontal part of duodenum
27. 十二指肠降部 descending part of duodenum

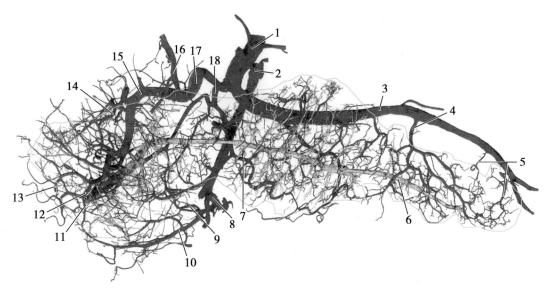

图 5-15　胰腺动脉和胰管的彩色铸型（前面观）
Colored resin corrosion cast for arteries of pancreas and pancreatic duct（anterior view）

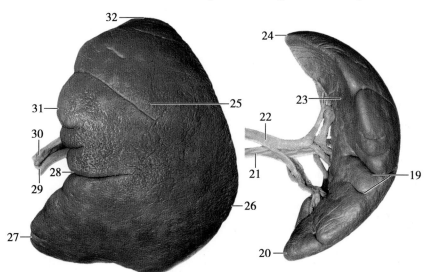

图 5-16　脾 Spleen

1. 腹腔干 celiac trunk
2. 肠系膜上动脉 superior mesenteric artery
3. 脾动脉 splenic artery
4. 胰大动脉 great pancreatic artery
5. 胰尾动脉 caudal pancreatic artery
6、11. 胰管 pancreatic duct
7. 胰下动脉 inferior pancreatic artery
8. 空肠动脉 jejunal artery
9、10. 胰十二指肠下动脉 inferior pancreaticoduodenal artery
12. 胰十二指肠前上动脉 anterior superior pancreaticoduodenal artery

13. 胃网膜右动脉 right gastro-epiploic artery
14. 胰十二指肠后上动脉 posterior superior pancreaticoduodenal artery
15. 胃十二指肠动脉 gastroduodenal artery
16. 肝固有动脉 proper hepatic artery
17. 肝总动脉 common hepatic artery
18. 胰背动脉 dorsal pancreatic artery
19、28. 脾切迹 notches of spleen

20、27. 脾前端 anterior extremity of spleen
21、29. 脾静脉 splenic vein
22、30. 脾动脉 splenic artery
23. 脾脏面 visceral surface of spleen
24、32. 脾后端 posterior extremity of spleen
25. 脾膈面 diaphragmatic surface of spleen
26. 脾下缘 inferior border of spleen
31. 脾上缘 superior border of spleen

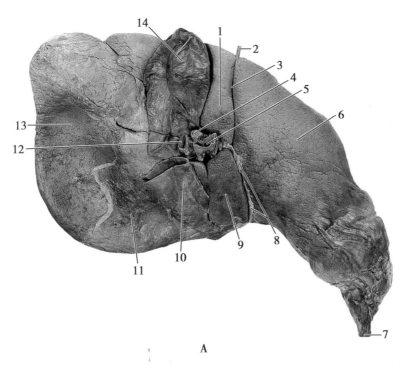

1. 肝方叶 quadrate lobe of liver
2. 肝圆韧带 round ligament of liver
3. 肝圆韧带裂 fissure for round ligament
4. 肝固有动脉 proper hepatic artery
5. 肝门静脉 hepatic portal vein
6、18. 肝左叶 left lobe of liver
7、19. 左三角韧带 left triangular ligament
8. 肝胃韧带 hepatogastric ligament
9. 肝尾状叶 caudate lobe of liver
10、29. 下腔静脉 inferior vena cava
11、22. 肝裸区 bare area of liver
12. 胆总管 common bile duct
13、24. 肝右叶 right lobe of liver
14. 胆囊 gallbladder

15. 主动脉 aorta
16. 食管 esophagus
17. 脾 spleen
20. 左冠状韧带后层 posterior layer of left coronary ligament
21. 左冠状韧带前层 anterior layer of left coronary ligament
23. 镰状韧带 falciform ligament
25. 右冠状韧带上层 superior layer of right coronary ligament
26. 右三角韧带 right triangular ligament
27. 膈 diaphragm
28. 肋膈隐窝 costodiaphragmatic recess

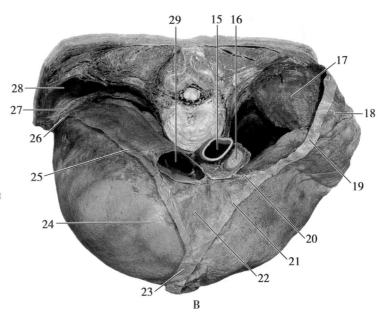

图 5-17 肝 Liver
A. 脏面 Visceral surface B. 膈面 Diaphragmatic surface

115

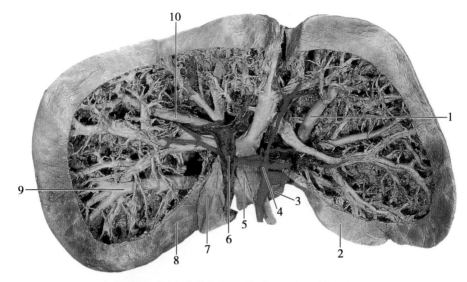

图 5-18 肝内血管和胆管（部分肝组织已被移除）
Blood vessels and biliary ducts within liver（portions of substance of liver have been removed）

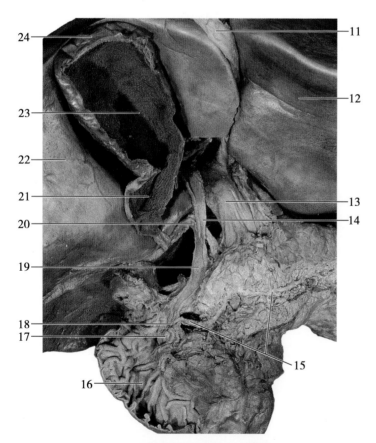

图 5-19 肝外胆道和胰管（胆囊和十二指肠已被切开）
**Extrahepatic biliary ducts and pancreatic duct
（gallbladder and duodenum have been opened）**

1、9、10. 肝静脉 hepatic vein

2、12. 肝左叶 left lobe of liver

3. 肝尾状叶 caudate lobe of liver

4. 肝固有动脉 proper hepatic artery

5、13. 肝门静脉 hepatic portal vein

6、14. 肝总管 common hepatic duct

7. 胆囊 gallbladder

8、22. 肝右叶 right lobe of liver

11. 肝圆韧带 round ligament of liver

15. 胰管 pancreatic duct

16. 十二指肠降部 descending part of duodenum

17. 十二指肠大乳头 major duodenal papilla

18. 肝胰腹壶 hepatopancreatic ampulla

19. 胆总管 common bile duct

20. 胆囊管 cystic duct

21. 胆囊颈 neck of gallbladder

23. 胆囊体 body of gallbladder

24. 胆囊底 fundus of gallbladder

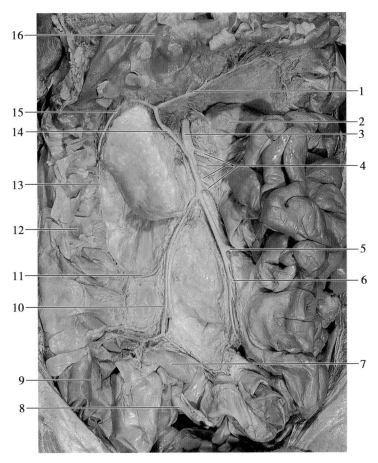

图 5-20　肠系膜上动脉（前面观）
Superior mesenteric artery（anterior view）

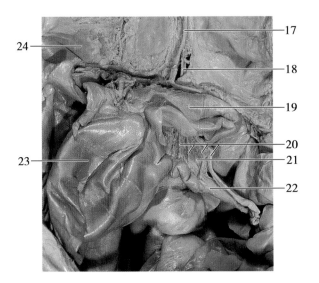

图 5-21　回结肠动脉（前面观）
Ileocolic artery（anterior view）

1. 中结肠动脉左支 left branch
   of middle colic artery
2. 十二指肠空肠曲 duodenojejunal flexure
3. 肠系膜上动脉 superior mesenteric artery
4、5. 空肠动脉 jejunal arteries
6. 回肠动脉 ileal artery
7、19. 回肠 ileum
8、22. 阑尾 vermiform appendix
9、23. 盲肠 cecum
10、17. 回结肠动脉 ileocolic artery
11. 右结肠动脉 right colic artery
12、24. 升结肠 ascending colon
13. 边缘动脉 marginal artery
14. 中结肠动脉 middle colic artery
15. 中结肠动脉右支 right branch
    of middle colic artery
16. 横结肠 transverse colon
18、20. 阑尾动脉、静脉 appendicular
        artery and vein
21. 阑尾系膜 mesoappendix

117

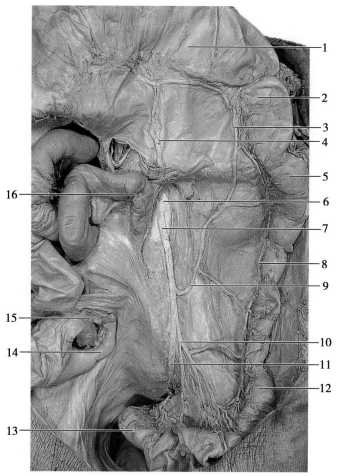

图 5-22 肠系膜下动脉（前面观）
Inferior mesenteric artery（anterior view）

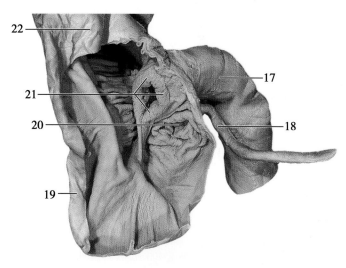

图 5-23 回盲部（前面观）
Ileocecal junction（anterior view）

1. 横结肠 transverse colon
2. 结肠左曲 left colic flexure
3、8. 边缘动脉 marginal artery
4. 中结肠动脉 middle colic artery
5. 降结肠 descending colon
6. 腹主动脉 abdominal aorta
7. 肠系膜下动脉 inferior mesenteric artery
9. 左结肠动脉 left colic artery
10. 乙状结肠动脉 sigmoid artery
11. 直肠上动脉 superior rectal artery
12. 乙状结肠 sigmoid colon
13. 直肠 rectum
14、18. 阑尾 vermiform appendix
15. 阑尾系膜 mesoappendix
16. 十二指肠空肠曲 duodenojejunal flexure
17. 回肠 ileum
19. 盲肠 cecum
20. 阑尾口 orifice of vermiform appendix
21. 回盲瓣 ileocecal valve
22. 升结肠 ascending colon

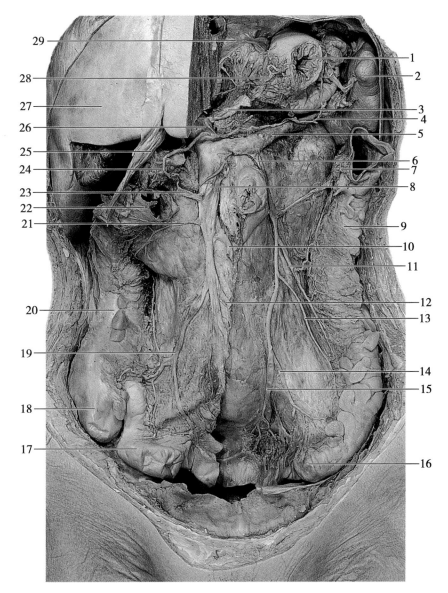

图 5-24 肝门静脉 (空肠、回肠、横结肠连同它们的系膜已除去)
Hepatic portal vein (jejunum, ileum, transverse colon and their mesentery have been removed)

1. 胃底 fundus of stomach
2. 脾 spleen
3. 胃左静脉 left gastric vein
4. 胃网膜左静脉 left gastroepiploic vein
5. 脾静脉 splenic vein
6. 肠系膜下静脉 inferior mesenteric vein
7. 结肠左曲 left colic flexure
8. 肠系膜上静脉 superior mesenteric vein
9. 降结肠 descending colon
10、12. 空肠静脉 jejunal veins
11. 左结肠静脉 left colic vein
13、14. 乙状结肠静脉 sigmoid veins
15. 直肠上静脉 superior rectal vein
16. 乙状结肠 sigmoid colon

17. 回肠 ileum
18. 盲肠 cecum
19. 回结肠静脉 ileocolic vein
20. 升结肠 ascending colon
21. 右结肠静脉 right colic vein
22. 结肠右曲 right colic flexure
23. 中结肠静脉 middle colic vein
24. 胃网膜右静脉 right gastroepiploic vein
25. 肝圆韧带 round ligament of liver
26. 肝门静脉 hepatic portal vein
27. 肝右叶 right lobe of liver
28. 胃底部静脉 veins of fundus of stomach
29. 食管腹段 abdominal part of esophagus

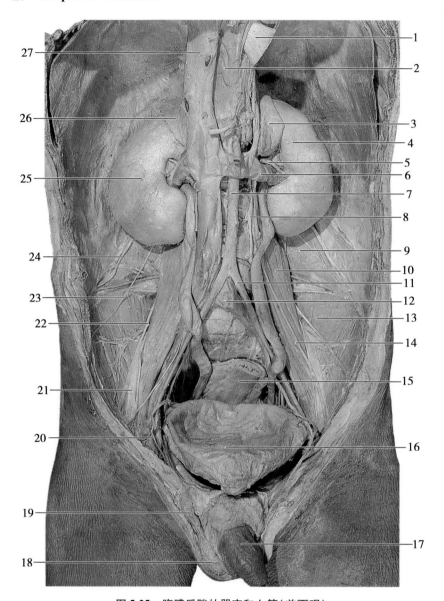

图 5-25　腹膜后隙的器官和血管(前面观)
Viscera and blood vessels within retroperitoneum(anterior view)

1. 食管腹段 abdominal part of esophagus
2. 膈 diaphragm
3. 左肾上腺 left suprarenal gland
4. 左肾 left kidney
5. 左肾动脉 left renal artery
6. 左肾静脉 left renal vein
7. 腹主动脉 abdominal aorta
8. 交感干腰节 lumbar ganglion of sympathetic trunk
9. 腰方肌 quadratus lumborum
10. 腰大肌 psoas major
11. 左髂总动脉 left common iliac artery
12. 左髂总静脉 left common iliac vein
13. 髂肌 iliacus
14. 生殖股神经 genitofemoral nerve

15. 直肠 rectum
16. 膀胱 urinary bladder
17. 阴茎 penis
18. 右侧睾丸 right testis
19. 右侧精索 right spermatic cord
20. 右侧输精管 right vas deferens
21. 生殖股神经 genitofemoral nerve
22. 股神经 femoral nerve
23. 股外侧皮神经 lateral femoral cutaneous nerve
24. 髂腹股沟神经 ilioinguinal nerve
25. 右肾 right kidney
26. 右肾上腺 right suprarenal gland
27. 下腔静脉 inferior vena cava

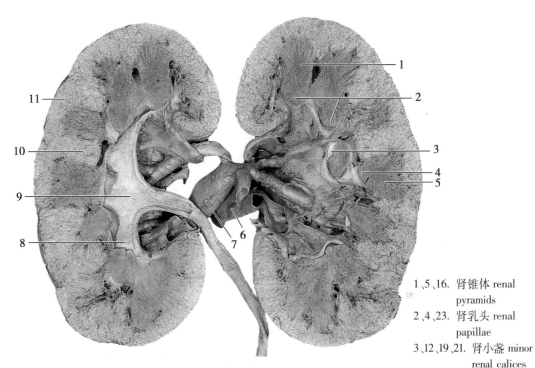

图 5-26　肾冠状切面
Coronary section of kidney

1、5、16. 肾锥体 renal
pyramids

2、4、23. 肾乳头 renal
papillae

3、12、19、21. 肾小盏 minor
renal calices

6. 肾静脉 renal vein

7. 肾动脉 renal artery

8、13、20. 肾大盏 major renal
calices

9、14、17. 肾盂 renal pelvis

10. 肾柱 renal column

11、22. 肾皮质 renal cortex

15、18. 输尿管 ureter

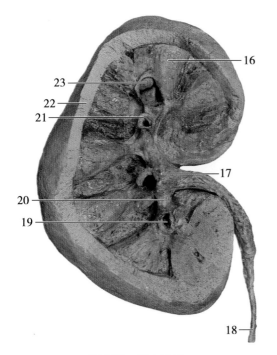

图 5-27　肾内结构
Internal structures of kidney

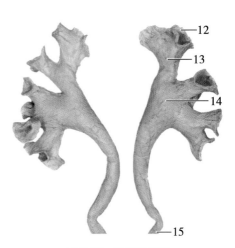

图 5-28　肾盏及肾盂
Renal calices and pelvis

121

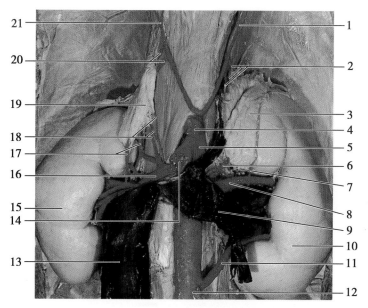

图 5-29　肾和肾上腺的动脉(前面观)
Arteries of kidneys and suprarenal glands(anterior view)

1. 左膈下动脉 left inferior phrenic artery
2、20. 肾上腺上动脉 superior suprarenal arteries
3. 左肾上腺 left suprarenal gland
4. 腹腔干 celiac trunk
5、12、26. 腹主动脉 abdominal aorta
6、18. 肾上腺中动脉 middle suprarenal arteries
7、17. 肾上腺下动脉 inferior suprarenal arteries
8、16. 肾动脉 renal artery
9. 左肾静脉 left renal vein
10. 左肾 left kidney
11、22、25. 副肾动脉 accessory renal artery
13. 下腔静脉 inferior vena cava
14. 肠系膜上动脉 superior mesenteric artery
15. 右肾 right kidney
19. 右肾上腺 right suprarenal gland
21. 右膈下动脉 right inferior phrenic artery

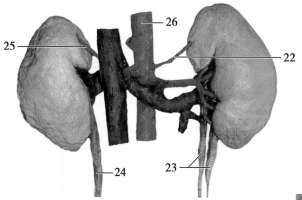

图 5-30　副肾动脉及双输尿管(前面观)
Accessory renal artery and double ureter (anterior view)

23、24、28、29、30. 输尿管 ureters
27. 马蹄肾 horseshoe kidney
31. 肾盂 renal pelvis
32. 腹腔神经节 celiac ganglia
33. 内脏大、小神经 greater and lesser splanchnic nerves

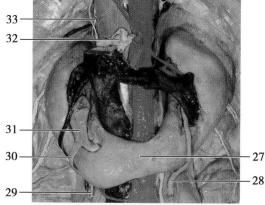

图 5-31　马蹄肾(前面观)
Horseshoe kidney(anterior view)

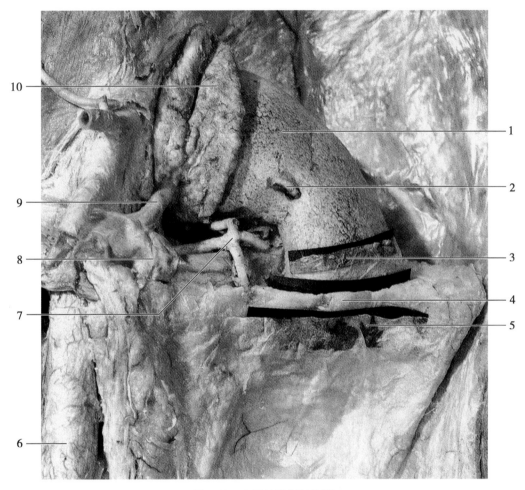

图 5-32　左肾被膜（前面观）
Coverings of left kidney（anterior view）

1. 肾 kidney
2. 副肾动脉 accessory renal artery
3. 肾纤维囊 fibrous capsule of kidney
4. 脂肪囊 adipose capsule
5. 肾筋膜 renal fascia
6. 腹主动脉 abdominal aorta
7. 左肾动脉 left renal artery
8. 左肾静脉 left renal vein
9. 左肾上腺静脉 left suprarenal vein
10. 左肾上腺 left suprarenal gland

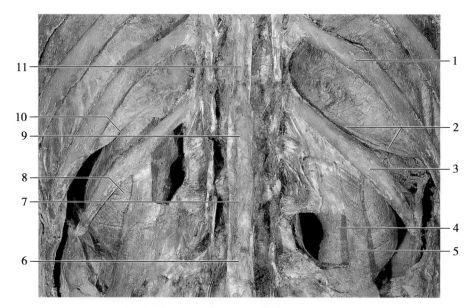

图 5-33 肾后面毗邻(后面观)
Structures related to posterior surface of kidney(posterior view)

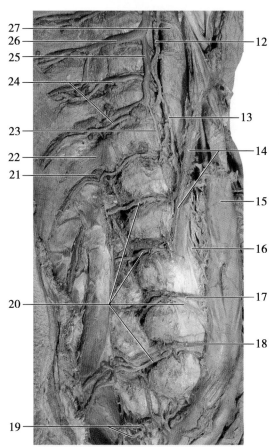

1. 第十一肋 eleventh rib
2、10. 胸膜下缘 inferior margin of pleura
3、22. 第十二肋 twelfth rib
4. 右肾 right kidney
5. 腰方肌 quadratus lumborum
6、7. 第二、第一腰椎棘突 spinous processes of second and first lumbar vertebrae
8. 左肾 left kidney
9、11. 第十二、第十一胸椎棘突 spinous processes of twelfth and eleventh vertebrae
12. 胸导管 thoracic duct
13. 乳糜池 cisterna chili
14. 右膈脚 right crus of diaphragm
15. 下腔静脉 inferior vena cava
16、17、18. 腰静脉 lumbar veins
19. 盆内静脉丛 venous plexuses of pelvis
20. 腰动脉 lumbar arteries
21. 肋下动脉 subcostal artery
23. 腰升静脉 ascending lumbar vein
24. 肋间后动脉 posterior intercostal arteries
25. 奇静脉 azygos vein
26. 肋间后静脉 posterior intercostal vein
27. 胸主动脉 thoracic aorta

图 5-34 腰动脉和腰静脉(右前外侧观)
Lumbar arteries and veins(right anterolateral view)

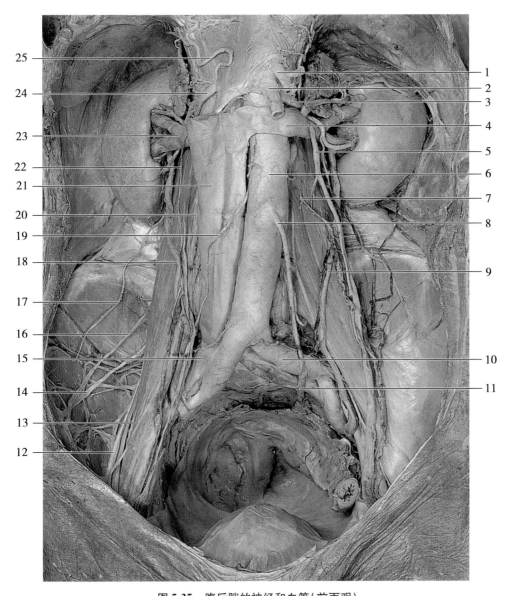

图 5-35　腹后隙的神经和血管（前面观）
Nerves and blood vessels within retroperitoneum（anterior view）

1. 腹腔干 celiac trunk
2. 肠系膜上动脉 superior mesenteric artery
3. 左肾动脉 left renal artery
4. 左肾静脉 left renal vein
5. 左睾丸静脉 left testicular vein
6. 腹主动脉 abdominal aorta
7. 左睾丸动脉 left testicular artery
8. 肠系膜下动脉 inferior mesenteric artery
9. 左输尿管 left ureter
10. 左髂总动脉 left common iliac artery
11. 直肠上动脉 superior rectal artery
12. 股神经 femoral nerve
13. 生殖股神经 genitofemoral nerve
14. 股外侧皮神经 lateral femoral cutaneous nerve
15. 右髂总静脉 right common iliac vein
16. 髂腹股沟神经 ilioinguinal nerve
17. 髂腹下神经 iliohypogastric nerve
18. 右输尿管 right ureter
19. 右睾丸动脉 right testicular artery
20. 腰大肌 psoas major
21. 下腔静脉 inferior vena cava
22. 右睾丸静脉 right testicular vein
23. 右肾静脉 right renal vein
24. 右肾动脉 right renal artery
25. 右膈下动脉 right inferior phrenic artery

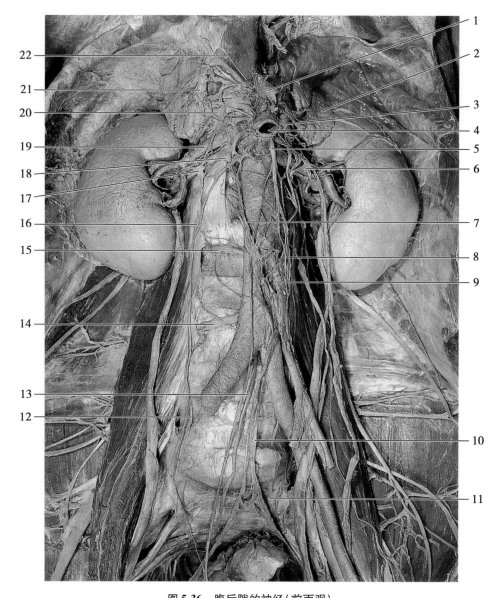

图 5-36　腹后隙的神经（前面观）
Nerves within retroperitoneum（anterior view）

1. 腹腔干 celiac trunk
2. 左肾上腺 left suprarenal gland
3、20. 腹腔神经节 celiac ganglia
4. 肠系膜上动脉 superior mesenteric artery
5. 肠系膜上丛 superior mesenteric plexus
6. 肾丛 renal plexus
7. 主动脉丛 aortic plexus
8. 肠系膜下丛 inferior mesenteric plexus
9. 肠系膜下动脉 inferior mesenteric artery
10. 上腹下丛 superior hypogastric plexus
11. 交感干骶节 sacral ganglia of sympathetic trunk
12、16. 交感干腰节 lumbar ganglia of sympathetic trunk
13. 骶正中动脉 median sacral artery
14、15. 腰动脉 lumbar arteries
17、18. 主动脉肾节 aorticorenal ganglia
19. 右肾动脉 right renal artery
21. 右肾上腺 right suprarenal gland
22. 膈神经 phrenic nerve

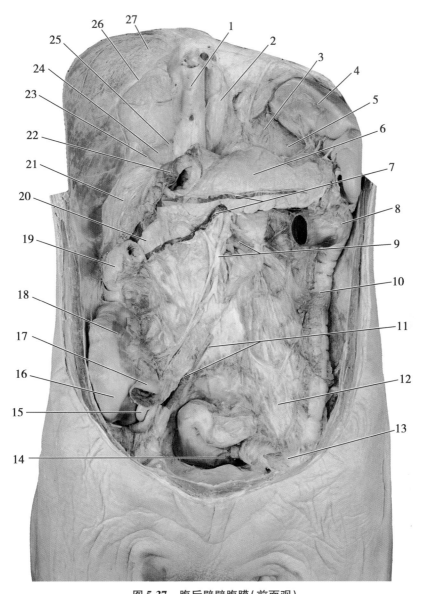

图 5-37 腹后壁壁腹膜(前面观)
Posterior parietal peritoneum(anterior view)

1. 下腔静脉 inferior vena cava
2. 腹主动脉 abdominal aorta
3. 左肾上腺 left suprarenal gland
4. 脾 spleen
5. 左肾上极 superior pole of left kidney
6. 胰体 body of pancreas
7. 横结肠系膜附着处(已切断)attachment of root of transverse mesocolon(has been cut)
8. 结肠左曲 left colic flexure
9. 肠系膜上动脉和静脉 superior mesenteric artery and vein
10. 降结肠 descending colon
11. 肠系膜附着处(已切断) attachment of root of mesentery(has been cut)
12. 乙状结肠系膜 sigmoid mesocolon
13. 乙状结肠 sigmoid colon
14. 直肠 rectum
15. 阑尾 vermiform appendix
16. 盲肠 cecum
17. 回肠 ileum
18. 升结肠 ascending colon
19. 结肠右曲 right colic flexure
20. 胰头 head of pancreas
21. 十二指肠降部 descending part of duodenum
22. 幽门 pylorus
23. 肝右冠状韧带下层 lower layer of right coronary ligament of liver
24. 右肾上极 superior pole of right kidney
25. 右肾上腺 right suprarenal gland
26. 肝右冠状韧带上层 upper layer of right coronary ligament of liver
27. 膈下表面 inferior surface of diaphragm

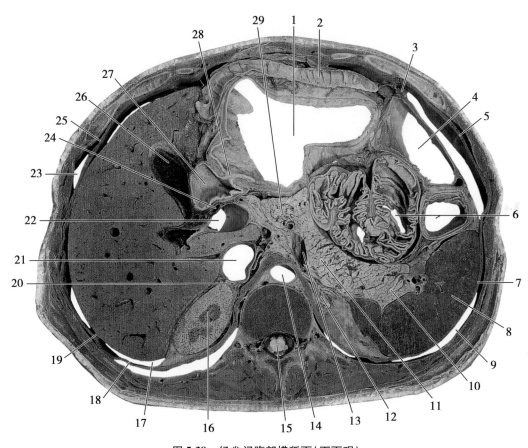

图 5-38　经幽门腹部横断面（下面观）
Transverse section through abdomen at level of pylorus(inferior view)

1. 胃 stomach
2. 回肠 ileum
3. 膈结肠韧带 phrenicocolic ligament
4. 结肠左曲 left colic flexure
5、7、18、25. 膈 diaphragm
6. 空肠 jejunum
8. 脾 spleen
9、23. 肋膈隐窝 costodiaphragmatic recesses
10. 胰尾 tail of pancreas
11. 胰体 body of pancreas
12. 左肾上腺 left suprarenal gland
13. 脾静脉 splenic vein
14. 腹主动脉 abdominal aorta

15. 脊髓 spinal cord
16. 右肾 right kidney
17. 肝肾隐窝（囊）hepatorenal recess(pouch)
19. 右三角韧带 right triangular ligament
20. 右肾上腺 right suprarenal gland
21. 下腔静脉 inferior vena cava
22. 肝门静脉 hepatic portal vein
24. 胆总管 common bile duct
26. 胆囊 gallbladder
27. 十二指肠上部 superior part of duodenum
28. 幽门口 pyloric orifice
29. 胰头 head of pancreas

第 6 章　盆与会阴

Chapter 6　Pelvis and Perineum

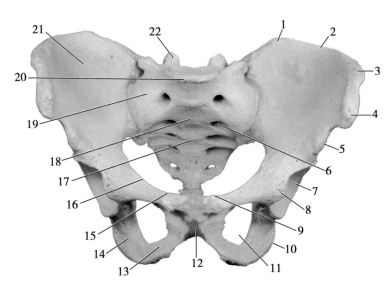

图 6-1　男性骨盆上口（上面观）
Superior pelvic aperture of male (superior view)

1. 髂后上棘 posterior superior iliac spine
2. 髂嵴 iliac crest
3. 髂结节 tubercle of iliac crest
4. 髂前上棘 anterior superior iliac spine
5. 髂前下棘 anterior inferior iliac spine
6. 骶前孔 anterior sacral foramina
7. 髋臼 acetabulum
8. 髂耻隆起 iliopubic eminence
9. 耻骨结节 pubic tubercle
10. 坐骨结节 ischial tuberosity
11. 闭孔 obturator foramen
12. 耻骨联合 pubic symphysis
13. 坐骨支 ramus of ischium
14. 坐骨体 body of ischium
15. 耻骨嵴 pubic crest
16. 弓状线 arcuate line
17. 横线 transverse line
18. 骶骨 sacrum
19. 骶翼 ala of sacrum
20. 骶岬 promontory of sacrum
21. 髂窝 iliac fossa
22. 骶骨上关节突 superior articular process of sacrum

1. 骶管裂孔 sacral hiatus
2. 尾骨 coccyx
3. 骶岬 promontory of sacrum
4. 坐骨大切迹 greater sciatic notch
5. 坐骨结节 ischial tuberosity
6. 髋臼 acetabulum
7. 闭孔 obturator foramen
8. 耻骨梳 pectin pubis
9. 耻骨结节 pubic tubercle
10. 耻骨联合 pubic symphysis
11. 耻骨体 body of pubis
12. 坐骨支 ramus of ischium
13. 髂前下棘 anterior inferior iliac spine
14. 髂结节 tubercle of iliac crest
15. 髂嵴 iliac crest
16. 骶前孔 anterior sacral foramina
17. 骶骨上关节突 superior articular process of sacrum

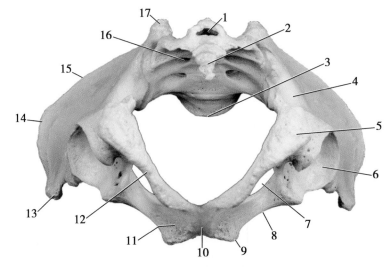

图 6-2　男性骨盆下口（下面观）
Inferior pelvic aperture of male (inferior view)

130

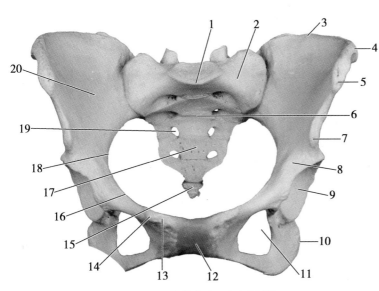

1. 骶岬 promontory of sacrum
2. 骶翼 ala of sacrum
3. 髂嵴 iliac crest
4. 髂结节 tubercle of iliac crest
5. 髂前上棘 anterior superior iliac spine
6. 横线 transverse line
7. 髂前下棘 anterior inferior iliac spine
8. 髂耻隆起 iliopubic eminence
9. 髋臼 acetabulum
10. 坐骨结节 ischial tuberosity
11. 闭孔 obturator foramen
12. 耻骨联合 pubic symphysis
13. 耻骨嵴 pubic crest
14. 耻骨结节 pubic tubercle
15. 尾骨 coccyx
16. 耻骨梳 pectin pubis
17. 骶骨 sacrum
18. 弓状线 arcuate line
19. 骶前孔 anterior sacral foramina
20. 髂翼 ala of ilium

图 6-3　女性骨盆上口(上面观)
Superior pelvic aperture of female(superior view)

1. 骶管裂孔 sacral hiatus
2. 骶角 sacral cornu
3. 髂后下棘 posterior inferior iliac spine
4. 尾骨 coccyx
5. 骶骨 sacrum
6. 坐骨棘 ischial spine
7. 坐骨结节 ischial tuberosity
8. 髋臼 acetabulum
9. 耻骨梳 pectin pubis
10. 耻骨结节 pubic tubercle
11. 耻骨嵴 pubic crest
12. 耻骨联合 pubic symphysis
13. 耻骨支 ramus of pubis
14. 坐骨支 ramus of ischium
15. 坐骨小切迹 lesser sciatic notch
16. 坐骨大切迹 greater sciatic notch
17. 骶翼 ala of sacrum
18. 骶岬 promontory of sacrum

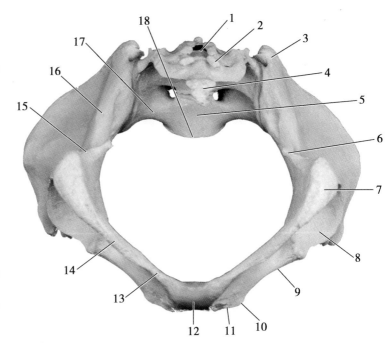

图 6-4　女性骨盆下口(下面观)
Inferior pelvic aperture of female(inferior view)

131

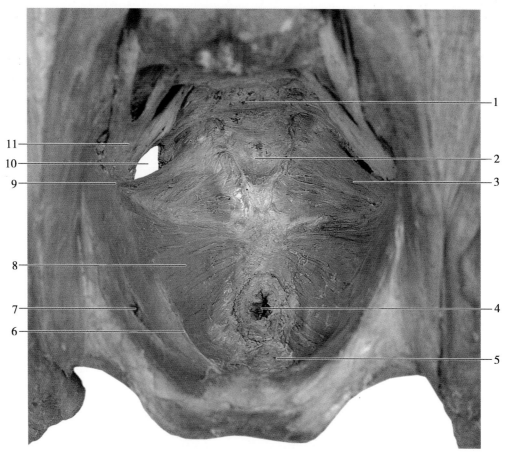

图 6-5 男性肛提肌（上面观）
Levator ani of male（superior view）

1. 骶骨 sacrum
2. 尾骨 coccyx
3. 尾骨肌 coccygeus
4. 直肠 rectum
5. 尿道膜部 membranous urethra
6. 肛提肌腱弓 tendinous arch of levator ani
7. 闭孔 obturator foramen
8. 肛提肌 levator ani
9. 坐骨棘 ischial spine
10. 坐骨大孔 greater sciatic foramen
11. 骶丛 sacral plexus

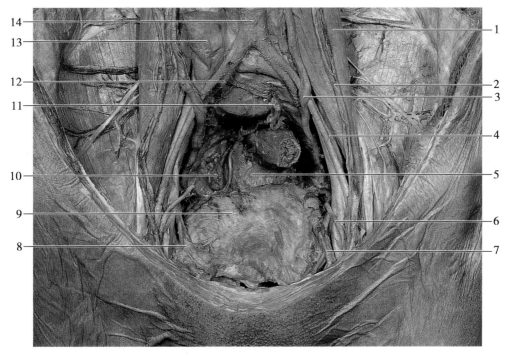

图 6-6　男性盆部(上面观)
Pelvis of male(superior view)

1. 腰大肌 psoas major
2. 睾丸动脉和静脉 testicular artery and vein
3. 输尿管 ureter
4. 髂外动脉和静脉 external iliac artery and vein
5. 直肠 rectum
6. 输精管 vas deferens
7. 腹壁下动脉和静脉 inferior epigastric artery and vein
8. 脐内侧制带 medial umbilical ligament
9. 膀胱 urinary bladder
10. 精囊 seminal vesicle
11. 直肠上动脉和静脉 superior rectal artery and vein
12. 髂内动脉 internal iliac artery
13. 下腔静脉 inferior vena cava
14. 腹主动脉 abdominal aorta

图 6-7　男性盆部正中矢状面 (右侧面观)
Median sagittal section of male pelvis
(right lateral view)

1. 直肠 rectum
2. 直肠膀胱陷凹 rectovesical pouch
3. 精囊 seminal vesicle
4. 前列腺中叶 median lobe of prostate
5. 射精管 ejaculatory duct
6. 前列腺后叶 posterior lobe of prostate
7. 尿生殖膈 urogenital diaphragm
8. 尿道球 bulb of penis
9. 阴囊中隔 septum of scrotum
10. 尿道海绵体部 penile urethra
11. 尿道膜部 membranous urethra
12. 前列腺前叶 anterior lobe of prostate
13. 尿道前列腺部 prostate urethra
14. 尿道内口 internal urethral orifice

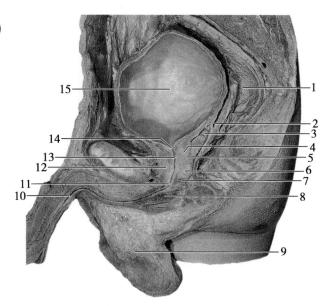

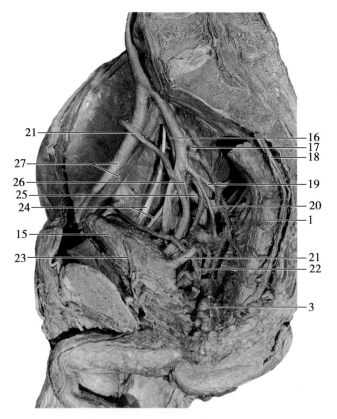

图 6-8　男性盆腔 (右侧面观)
Pelvic cavity of male (right lateral view)

15. 膀胱 urinary bladder
16. 髂内动脉、静脉 internal iliac artery and vein
17. 臀上动脉 superior gluteal artery
18. 直肠上动脉、静脉 superior rectal artery and vein
19. 阴部内动脉 internal pudendal artery
20. 直肠下动脉 inferior rectal artery
21. 输尿管 ureter
22. 输精管 vas deferens
23. 膀胱上动脉 superior vesical artery
24. 闭孔神经、动脉 obturator nerve and artery
25. 臀下动脉 inferior gluteal artery
26. 膀胱下动脉 inferior vesical artery
27. 髂外动脉、静脉 external iliac artery and vein

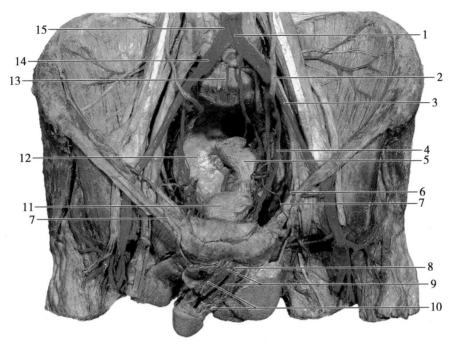

图 6-9　男性盆部动脉（上面观）
Arteries of male pelvis（superior view）

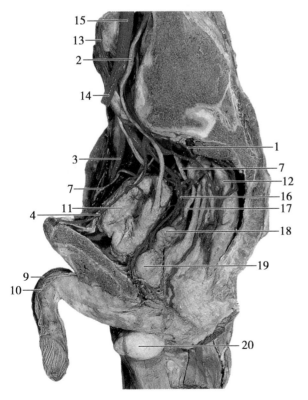

图 6-10　男性盆部动脉（右侧面观）
Arteries of male pelvis（right lateral view）

1. 直肠上动脉 superior rectal artery
2. 输尿管 ureter
3. 髂外动脉 external iliac artery
4. 脐动脉 umbilical artery
5. 乙状结肠 sigmoid colon
6. 腹壁下动脉闭孔支（副闭孔动脉）obturator branch of inferior epigastric artery（accessory obturator artery）
7. 输精管 vas deferens
8. 阴茎背深静脉 deep dorsal vein of penis
9. 阴茎背动脉 dorsal artery of penis
10. 阴茎背神经 dorsal nerve of penis
11. 膀胱 urinary bladder
12. 直肠 rectum
13. 骶正中动脉 median sacral artery
14. 髂总动脉 common iliac artery
15. 腹主动脉 abdominal aorta
16. 膀胱下动脉 inferior vesical artery
17. 输精管壶腹 ampulla of vas deferens
18. 精囊 seminal vesicle
19. 前列腺 prostate
20. 睾丸 testis

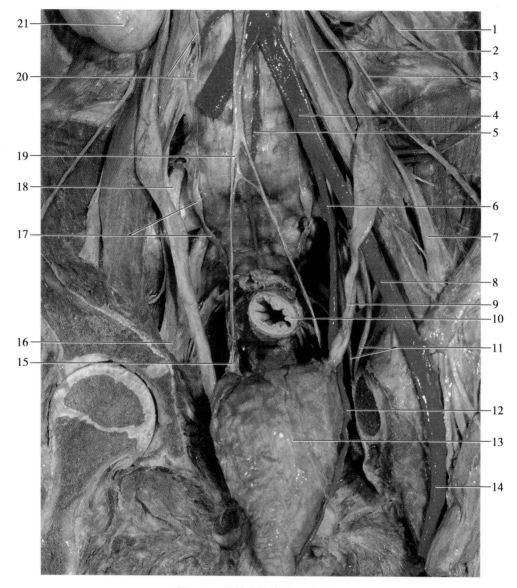

图 6-11 男性盆部神经(上面观)
Nerves of male pelvis(superior view)

1. 髂腹股沟神经 ilioinguinal nerve
2. 生殖股神经 genitofemoral nerve
3. 股外侧皮神经 lateral femoral cutaneous nerve
4. 髂总动脉 common iliac artery
5. 骶正中动脉 median sacral artery
6. 髂内动脉 internal iliac artery
7. 股神经 femoral nerve
8. 髂外动脉 external iliac artery
9. 输尿管 ureter
10. 直肠 rectum
11. 闭孔神经、动脉 obturator nerve and artery

12. 脐动脉 umbilical artery
13. 膀胱 urinary bladder
14. 股动脉 femoral artery
15. 下腹下丛 inferior hypogastric plexus
16. 骶丛 sacral plexus
17. 交感干骶节 sacral ganglia of sympathetic trunk
18. 腰骶干 lumbosacral trunk
19. 上腹下丛 superior hypogastric plexus
20. 交感干腰节 lumbar ganglion of sympathetic trunk
21. 肾 kidney

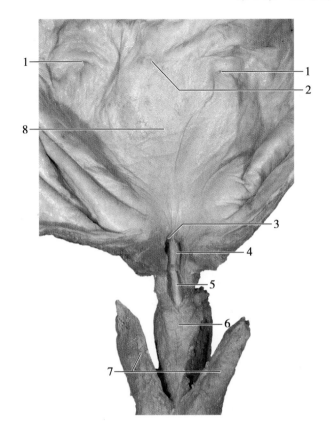

图 6-12 男性膀胱（内面观）
Male urinary bladder（internal view）
1. 输尿管口 ureteric orifice
2. 输尿管间襞 interureteric fold
3. 尿道内口 internal urethral orifice
4. 精阜 seminal colliculus
5. 尿道嵴 urethral crest
6. 尿道球 bulb of penis
7. 阴茎脚 crus of penis
8. 膀胱三角 trigone of urinary bladder

图 6-13 前列腺和精囊（后面观）
Prostate and seminal vesicle
（posterior view）
1. 输精管 vas deferens
2. 输尿管 ureter
3. 精囊 seminal vesicle
4. 输精管壶腹 ampulla of vas deferens
5. 精囊排泄管 excretory duct of seminal
   vesicle
6. 射精管 ejaculatory duct
7. 阴茎脚 crus of penis
8. 尿道球 bulb of penis
9. 前列腺 prostate
10. 膀胱 urinary bladder

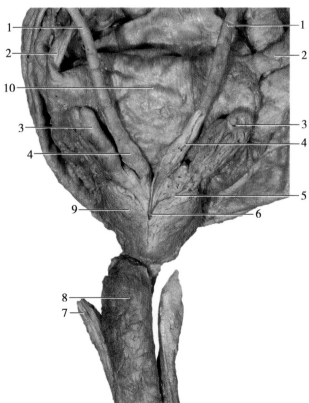

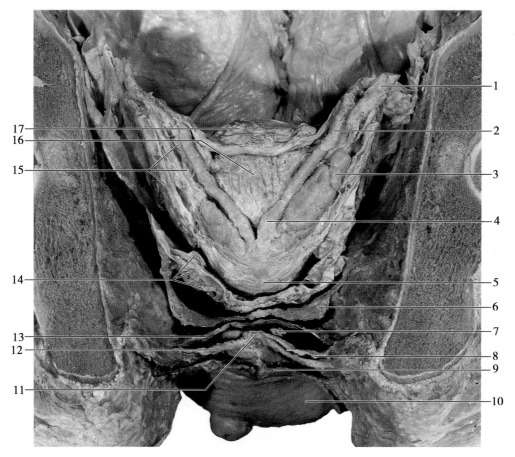

图 6-14　男性膀胱底(后面观)
Fundus of male urinary bladder(posterior view)

1. 输尿管 ureter
2. 输精管 vas deferens
3. 精囊 seminal vesicle
4. 输精管壶腹 ampulla of vas deferens
5. 前列腺 prostate
6. 肛提肌(盆膈) levator ani(pelvic diaphragm)
7. 尿道球腺 bulbo-urethral gland
8. 尿生殖膈下筋膜(会阴膜) inferior fascia of urogenital diaphragm(perineal membrane)
9. 会阴浅筋膜 superficial fascia of perineum
10. 阴囊 scrotum
11. 会阴体(会阴中心腱) perineal body(perineal central tendon)
12. 会阴浅横肌 superficial transverse perineal muscle
13. 会阴深横肌 deep transverse perineal muscle
14. 前列腺静脉丛 prostatic venous plexus
15. 膀胱静脉丛 vesical venous plexus
16. 膀胱 urinary bladder
17. 腹膜 peritoneum

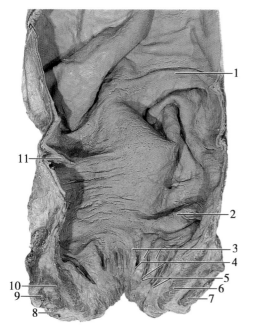

图 6-15　直肠(内面观)
Rectum(internal view)
1. 上直肠横襞 superior transverse rectal fold
2. 下直肠横襞 inferior transverse rectal fold
3. 肛柱 anal columns
4. 肛窦 anal sinuses
5. 肛瓣 anal valves
6. 肛门内括约肌 internal ani sphincter
7. 肛门外括约肌 external ani sphincter
8. 肛门外括约肌皮下部 subcutaneous part of external ani sphincter
9. 肛门外括约肌浅部 superficial part of external ani sphincter
10. 肛门外括约肌深部 deep part of external ani sphincter
11. 中直肠横襞 middle transverse rectal fold

1. 输尿管 ureter
2. 输精管 vas deferens
3. 精囊腺 seminal vesicle
4. 前列腺 prostate
5. 膀胱颈 neck of urinary bladder
6. 膀胱底 base of urinary bladder
7. 膀胱体 body of urinary bladder
8. 膀胱尖 apex of urinary bladder
9. 脐正中韧带(闭合的尿囊管) median umbilical ligament(obliterated allantoic canal)

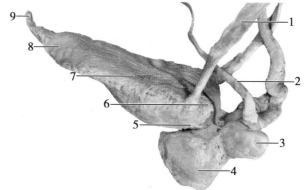

图 6-16　膀胱、前列腺和精囊腺(右侧面观)
Urinary bladder,prostate and seminal vesicle(right lateral view)

图 6-17　前列腺横断面
Transverse section of prostate
1. 前列腺前叶 anterior lobe of prostate
2. 前列腺中叶 median lobe of prostate
3. 尿道前列腺部 prostate urethra
4. 射精管 ejaculatory duct
5. 精囊腺 seminal vesicle
6. 前列腺后叶 posterior lobe of prostate
7. 尿道嵴 urethral crest
8. 前列腺侧叶 lateral lobe of prostate

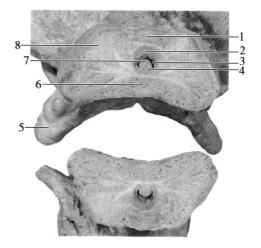

139

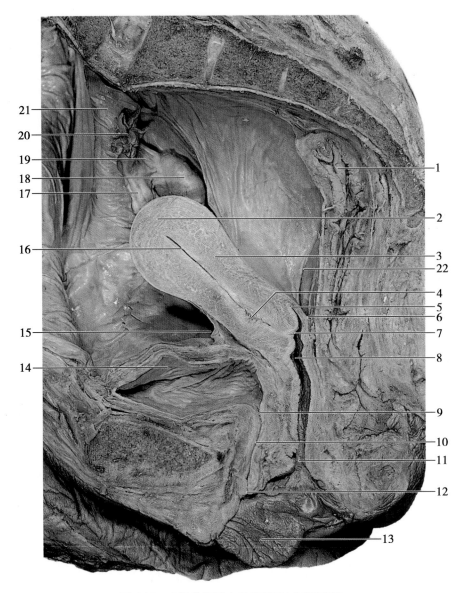

图 6-18　女性盆部正中矢状剖面（右侧面观）
Median sagittal section of female pelvis（right lateral view）

1. 直肠 rectum
2. 子宫底 fundus of uterus
3. 子宫体 body of uterus
4. 子宫颈管 canal of cervix uteri
5. 阴道穹后部 posterior fornix of vagina
6. 直肠子宫陷凹 rectouterine pouch
7. 宫颈外口 external os of cervix uteri
8. 阴道 vagina
9. 尿道内口 internal urethral orifice
10. 尿道 urethra
11. 阴道口 vaginal opening

12. 尿道外口 external urethral orifice
13. 小阴唇 labium minus
14. 膀胱 urinary bladder
15. 膀胱子宫陷凹 vesicouterine pouch
16. 子宫腔 cavity of uterus
17. 输卵管 uterine tube
18. 卵巢 ovary
19. 卵巢系膜 mesovarium
20. 输卵管伞 fimbriae of uterine tube
21. 卵巢悬韧带 suspensory ligament of ovary
22. 直肠子宫襞 rectouterine fold

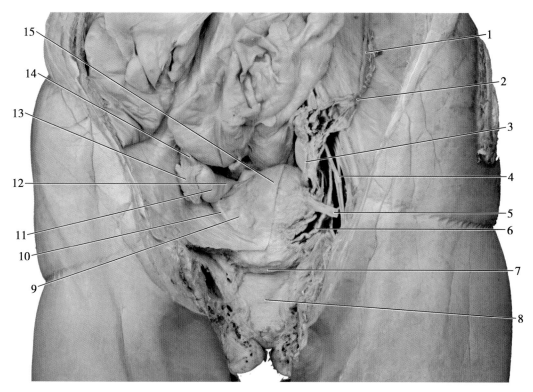

图 6-19 卵巢和子宫(前面观,膀胱和左侧半盆腔腹膜已移除)
Ovary and uterus(anterior view,urinary bladder and left half of
peritoneum has been removed)

1. 输尿管 ureter
2. 卵巢动脉和静脉 ovarian artery and vein
3. 输卵管 uterine tube
4. 闭孔神经、动脉和静脉 obturator nerve,artery and vein
5. 子宫圆韧带 round ligament of uterus
6. 子宫动脉(跨输尿管前方处)uterine artery(crosses above and in front of ureter)
7. 宫颈外口 external os of cervix uteri
8. 阴道后壁(前壁已移除)posterior wall of vagina(anterior wall has been removed)
9. 子宫阔韧带后层 posterior layer of broad ligament
10. 子宫阔韧带上缘 superior margin of broad ligament
11. 卵巢 ovary
12. 卵巢下端 inferior end of ovary
13. 输卵管伞 fimbriae of uterine tube
14. 卵巢悬韧带 suspensory ligament of ovary
15. 子宫 uterus

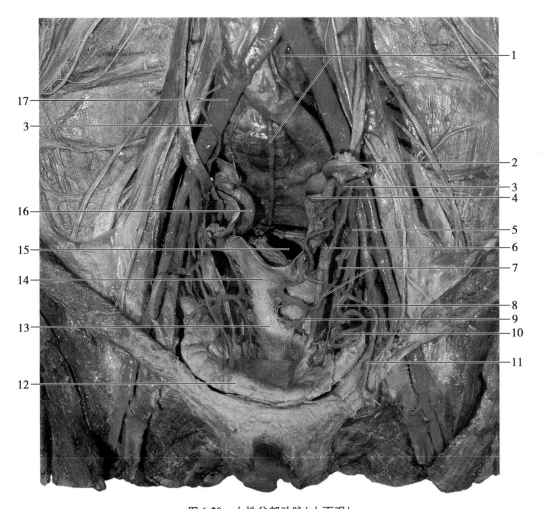

图 6-20　女性盆部动脉(上面观)
Arteries of female pelvis(superior view)

1. 骶正中动脉 median sacral artery
2. 输卵管伞 fimbriae of uterine tube
3. 卵巢动脉 ovarian artery
4. 输卵管 uterine tube
5. 髂内动脉 internal iliac artery
6. 输尿管 ureter
7. 子宫动脉 uterine artery
8. 膀胱下动脉 inferior vesical artery
9. 阴道动脉 vaginal artery
10. 脐动脉 umbilical artery
11. 子宫圆韧带 round ligament of uterus
12. 膀胱 urinary bladder
13. 子宫颈 neck of uterus
14. 子宫体 body of uterus
15. 直肠 rectum
16. 卵巢 ovary
17. 髂总动脉、静脉 common iliac artery and vein

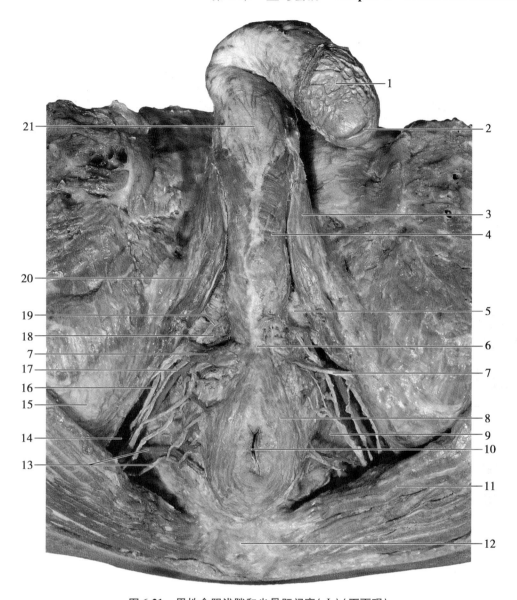

图 6-21　男性会阴浅隙和坐骨肛门窝（Ⅰ）（下面观）
Superficial perineal space and ischioanal fossa of male（Ⅰ）（inferior view）

1. 阴茎头 glans of penis
2. 尿道外口 external urethral orifice
3. 坐骨海绵体肌 ischiocavernosus
4. 球海绵体肌 bulbospongiosus
5. 尿生殖膈下筋膜（会阴膜）inferior fascia of urogenital diaphragm（perineal membrane）
6. 会阴体（会阴中心腱）perineal body（perineal central tendon）
7. 会阴浅横肌 superficial transverse perineal muscle
8. 肛门外括约肌 external ani sphincter
9. 肛提肌 levator ani
10. 肛门 anus
11. 臀大肌 gluteus maximus
12. 尾骨 coccyx
13. 肛神经、动脉 anal nerve and artery
14. 坐骨肛门窝 ischioanal fossa
15. 坐骨结节 ischial tuberosity
16. 阴茎背神经 dorsal nerve of penis
17. 会阴神经、动脉 perineal nerve and artery
18. 会阴深横肌 deep transverse perineal muscle
19. 阴囊后神经 posterior scrotal nerve
20. 耻骨弓 pubic arch
21. 阴茎体 body of penis

143

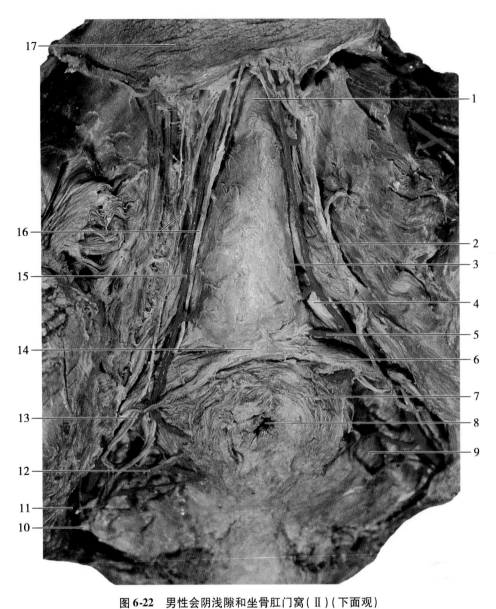

图 6-22 男性会阴浅隙和坐骨肛门窝(Ⅱ)(下面观)
Superficial perineal space and ischioanal fossa of male(Ⅱ)(inferior view)

1. 尿道海绵体 corpus spongiosum
2. 坐骨海绵体肌 ischiocavernosus
3. 球海绵体肌 bulbospongiosus
4. 尿生殖膈下筋膜(会阴膜) inferior fascia of urogenital diaphragm(perineal membrane)
5. 尿道球动脉 urethral bulbar artery
6. 会阴浅横肌 superficial transverse perineal muscle
7. 肛门外括约肌 external ani sphincter
8. 肛门 anus
9. 肛提肌 levator ani
10. 阴部神经 pudendal nerve
11. 阴部内动脉 internal pudendal artery
12. 肛神经、动脉 anal nerve and artery
13. 会阴神经、动脉 perineal nerve and artery
14. 会阴体(会阴中心腱) perineal body (perineal central tendon)
15. 阴囊后动脉 posterior scrotal artery
16. 阴囊后神经 posterior scrotal nerve
17. 阴囊 scrotum

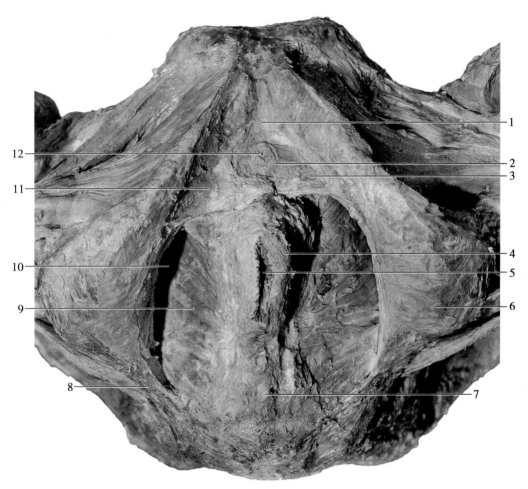

图 6-23　男性会阴深隙和坐骨肛门窝（下面观）
Deep perineal space and ischioanal fossa of male（inferior view）

1. 尿生殖膈下筋膜（会阴膜）inferior fascia of urogenital diaphragm（perineal membrane）
2. 尿道外括约肌 external urethral sphincter
3. 会阴深横肌 deep transverse perineal muscle
4. 肛门外括约肌 external ani sphincter
5. 肛门 anus
6. 坐骨结节 ischial tuberosity
7. 尾骨 coccyx
8. 骶结节韧带 sacrotuberous ligament
9. 肛提肌 levator ani
10. 坐骨肛门窝 ischioanal fossa
11. 会阴浅横肌 superficial transverse perineal muscle
12. 尿道膜部 membranous urethra

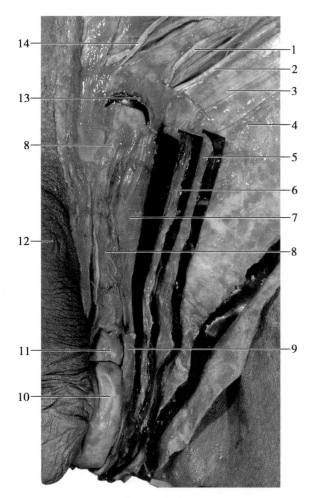

图 6-24 睾丸和精索被膜(前面观)
Testis and tunicae of spermatic cord (anterior view)

1. 髂腹股沟神经 ilioinguinal nerve
2. 腹股沟韧带 inguinal ligament
3. 腹外斜肌腱膜 aponeurosis of obliquus externus abdominis
4. 浅筋膜 superficial fascia
5. 精索外筋膜 external spermatic fascia
6. 提睾肌筋膜 cremasteric fascia
7. 精索内筋膜 internal spermatic fascia
8. 精索 spermatic cord
9. 睾丸鞘膜壁层 parietal layer of tunica vaginalis
10. 睾丸 testis
11. 附睾 epididymis
12. 阴茎 penis
13. 腹股沟管浅环 superficial inguinal ring
14. 髂腹下神经 iliohypogastric nerve

图 6-25 阴囊层次(前面观)
Layers of scrotum(anterior view)

1. 皮肤 skin
2. 肉膜 dartos coat
3. 精索外筋膜 external spermatic fascia
4. 提睾肌筋膜 cremasteric fascia
5. 精索内筋膜 internal spermatic fascia
6. 睾丸鞘膜壁层 parietal layer of tunica vaginalis
7. 睾丸 testis
8. 精索 spermatic cord

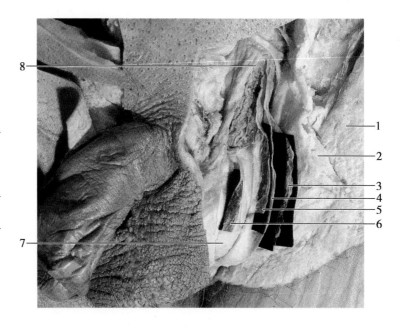

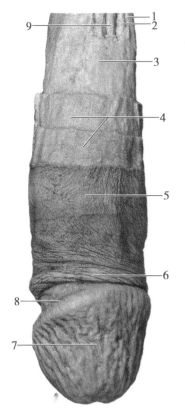

图 6-26　阴茎层次（背侧观）
Layers of penis（dorsal view）

1. 阴茎背神经 dorsal nerve of penis
2. 阴茎背动脉 dorsal artery of penis
3. 阴茎深筋膜 deep fascia of penis
4. 阴茎浅筋膜 superficial fascia of penis
5. 皮肤 skin
6. 阴茎包皮 prepuce of penis
7. 阴茎头 glans of penis
8. 阴茎颈 neck of penis
9. 阴茎背深静脉 deep dorsal vein of penis

图 6-27　阴茎勃起组织（腹侧观）
Erectile tissues of penis（ventral view）

1. 尿道球 bulb of penis
2. 阴茎脚 crus of penis
3. 尿道海绵体 corpus spongiosum
4. 阴茎头 glans of penis
5. 阴茎海绵体 corpus cavernosum
6. 阴茎背深静脉 deep dorsal vein of penis
7. 阴茎深动脉 deep artery of penis
8. 尿道 urethra
9. 海绵体白膜 tunica albuginea

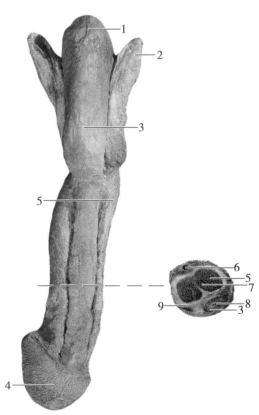

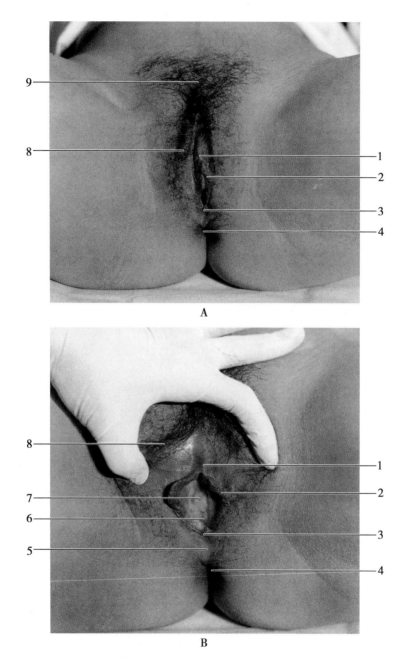

图 6-28　女性外生殖器 External genital organs of female
A. 下面观 Inferior view　B. 大阴唇被推向两侧 labia majora
are pulled to both sides

1. 阴蒂头及阴蒂包皮 glans clitoris and prepuce of clitoris
2. 小阴唇 labium minus
3. 阴唇系带 frenulum of clitoris
4. 肛门 anus
5. 唇后连合（覆盖会阴体）posterior commissure
　（overlies perineal body）
6. 阴道口 vaginal opening
7. 尿道外口 external urethral orifice
8. 大阴唇 labium majus
9. 阴阜 mons pubis

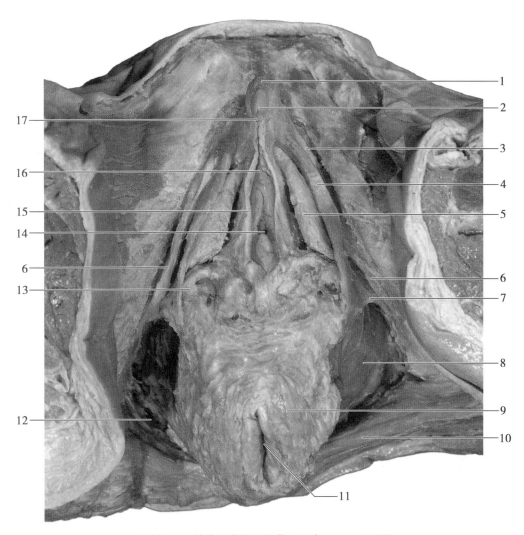

图 6-29　女性会阴浅隙和坐骨肛门窝（Ⅰ）（下面观）
Superficial perineal space and ischioanal fossa of female（Ⅰ）（inferior view）

1. 阴蒂海绵体 corpus cavernosum
2. 阴蒂头及阴蒂包皮 glans clitoris and prepuce of clitoris
3. 阴蒂脚 crus of clitoris
4. 球海绵体肌 bulbospongiosus
5. 前庭球 bulb of vestibule
6. 坐骨海绵体肌 ischiocavernosus
7. 会阴浅横肌 superficial transverse perineal muscle
8. 肛提肌 levator ani
9. 肛门外括约肌 external ani sphincter
10. 臀大肌 gluteus maximus
11. 肛门 anus
12. 坐骨肛门窝 ischioanal fossa
13. 前庭大腺 greater vestibular gland
14. 阴道口 vaginal opening
15. 小阴唇 labium minus
16. 尿道外口 external urethral orifice
17. 阴蒂系带 frenulum of clitoris

149

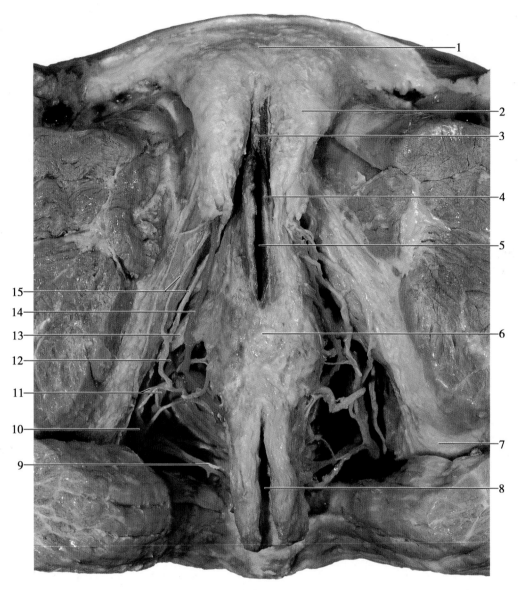

图 6-30　女性会阴浅隙和坐骨肛门窝（Ⅱ）（下面观）
Superficial perineal space and ischioanal fossa of female（Ⅱ）（inferior view）

1. 阴阜 mons pubis
2. 大阴唇 labium majus
3. 阴蒂头 glans clitoris
4. 小阴唇 labium minus
5. 阴道口 vaginal opening
6. 会阴体（会阴中心腱）perineal body（perineal central tendon）
7. 坐骨结节 ischial tuberosity

8. 肛门 anus
9. 肛神经、动脉 anal nerve and artery
10. 阴部神经 pudendal nerve
11. 会阴神经、动脉 perineal nerve and artery
12. 阴蒂深动脉 deep artery of clitoris
13. 会阴浅横肌 superficial transverse perineal muscle
14. 阴唇后动脉 posterior labial artery
15. 阴唇后神经 posterior labial nerve

第 7 章　背

Chapter 7　Back

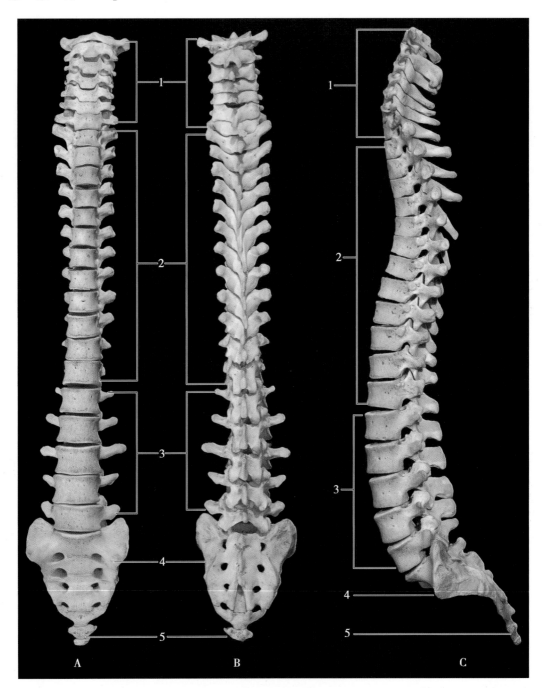

图 7-1　脊柱 Vertebral column

A. 前面观 Anterior view　B. 后面观 Posterior view　C. 侧面观 Lateral view

1. 颈椎 cervical vertebrae
2. 胸椎 thoracic vertebrae
3. 腰椎 lumbar vertebrae
4. 骶骨 sacrum
5. 尾骨 coccyx

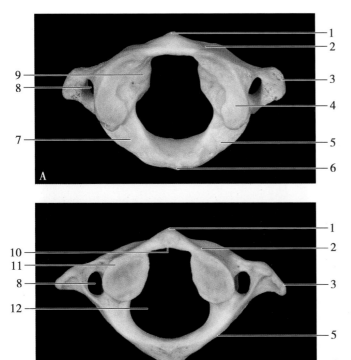

图 7-2 寰椎 Atlas

A. 上面观 Superior view
B. 下面观 Inferior view

1. 前结节 anterior tubercle
2. 前弓 anterior arch
3. 横突 transverse process
4. 上关节面 superior articular facet
5. 后弓 posterior arch
6. 后结节 posterior tubercle
7. 椎动脉沟 groove for vertebral artery
8. 横突孔 foramen transversarium
9. 侧块 lateral mass
10. 齿突面 facet for dens
11. 下关节面 inferior articular facet
12. 椎孔 vertebral foramen

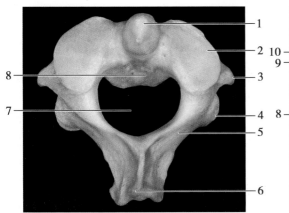

图 7-3 枢椎(上面观)
Axis(superior view)

1. 齿突 dens of axis
2. 上关节面 superior articular facet
3. 横突 transverse process
4. 下关节突 inferior articular process
5. 椎弓板 lamina of vertebral arch
6. 棘突 spinous process
7. 椎孔 vertebral foramen
8. 椎体 vertebral body

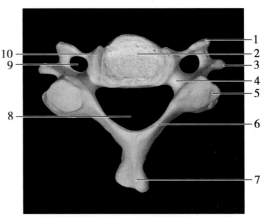

图 7-4 颈椎(上面观)
A cervical vertebra(superior view)

1. 横突前结节 anterior tubercle of transverse process
2. 椎体 vertebral body
3. 横突后结节 posterior tubercle of transverse process
4. 椎弓根 pedicle of vertebral arch
5. 上关节面 superior articular facet
6. 椎弓板 lamina of vertebral arch
7. 棘突 spinous process
8. 椎孔 vertebral foramen
9. 横突孔 foramen transversarium
10. 椎体钩 uncus of vertebral body

153

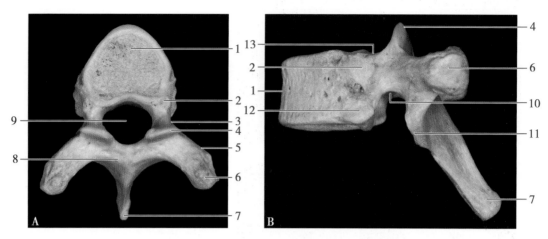

图 7-5 胸椎 A thoracic vertebra

A. 上面观（Superior view） B. 侧面观（Lateral view）

1. 椎体 vertebral body
2. 上肋凹 superior costal facet
3. 椎弓根 pedicle of vertebral arch
4. 上关节突 superior articular process
5. 横突 transverse process
6. 横突肋凹 costal facet of transverse process
7. 棘突 spinous process

8. 椎弓板 lamina of vertebral arch
9. 椎孔 vertebral foramen
10. 椎下切迹 inferior vertebral notch
11. 下关节突 inferior articular process
12. 下肋凹 inferior costal facet
13. 椎上切迹 superior vertebral notch

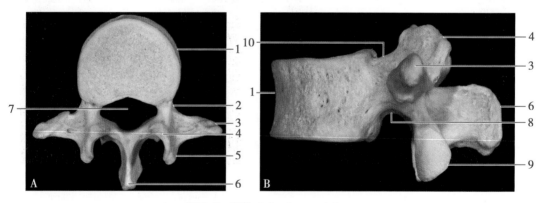

图 7-6 腰椎 A lumbar vertebra

A. 上面观（Superior view） B. 侧面观（Lateral view）

1. 椎体 vertebral body
2. 椎弓根 pedicle of vertebral arch
3. 横突 transverse process
4. 上关节突 superior articular process
5. 乳突 mammillary process

6. 棘突 spinous process
7. 椎孔 vertebral foramen
8. 椎下切迹 inferior vertebral notch
9. 下关节突 inferior articular process
10. 椎上切迹 superior vertebral notch

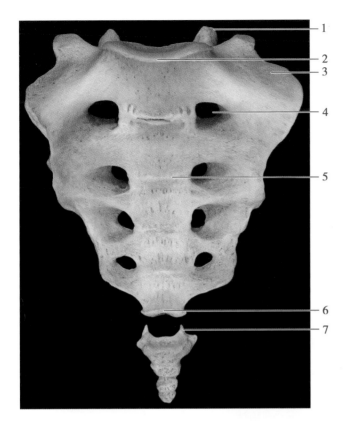

图 7-7 骶骨和尾骨(前面观)
Sacrum and coccyx(anterior view)
1. 上关节突 superior articular process
2. 骶岬 promontory of sacrum
3. 骶翼 ala of sacrum
4. 骶前孔 anterior sacral foramina
5. 横线 transverse line
6. 骶骨尖 apex of sacrum
7. 尾骨角 coccygeal cornu

图 7-8 骶骨和尾骨(后面观)
Sacrum and coccyx(posterior view)
1. 上关节突 superior articular facet
2. 骶管 sacral canal
3. 骶粗隆 sacral tuberosity
4. 耳状面 auricular surface
5. 骶正中嵴 median sacral crest
6. 骶外侧嵴 lateral sacral crest
7. 骶后孔 posterior sacral foramen
8. 骶中间嵴 intermediate sacral crest
9. 骶管裂孔 sacral hiatus
10. 骶角 sacral cornu
11. 尾骨角 coccygeal cornu

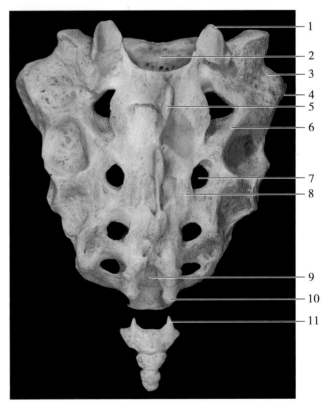

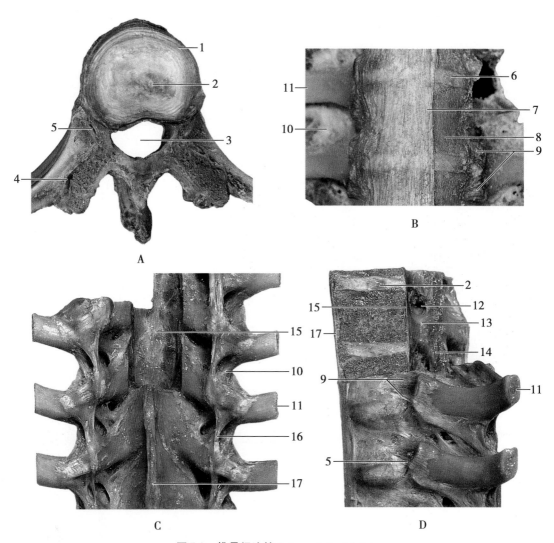

图 7-9 椎骨间连接 Intervertebral joints

A. 上面观 Superior view B. 前面观 Anterior view
C. 后面观 Posterior view D. 侧面观 Lateral view

1. 纤维环 anulus fibrosus
2. 髓核 nucleus pulposus
3. 椎孔 vertebral foramen
4. 肋横突关节 costotransverse joint
5. 肋头关节 joint of costal head
6. 椎间盘 intervertebral disc
7. 前纵韧带 anterior longitudinal ligament
8. 椎体 vertebral body
9. 辐状韧带 radiate ligament
10. 肋横突上韧带 superior costotransverse ligament
11. 肋骨 rib
12. 椎间孔 intervertebral foramen
13. 椎弓板 lamina of vertebral arch
14. 黄韧带 ligamentum flavum
15. 后纵韧带 posterior longitudinal ligament
16. 横突间韧带 intertransverse ligament
17. 棘上韧带 supraspinal ligament

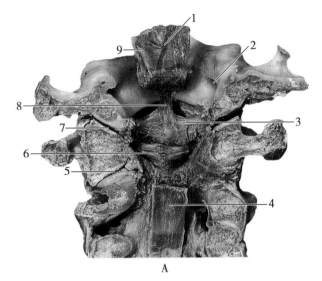

A

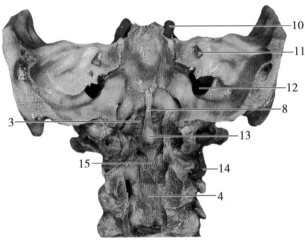

图 7-10 颅骨与椎骨连接
Joints of the skull and vertebra

　A. 后面观(覆膜已切断并上翻)
Posterior view(membrana tectoria has
　been cut and reflected upward)

　B. 后面观(覆膜已被移除) Posterior
　view(membrana tectoria has
　been removed)

　C. 侧面观 Lateral view

1. 上纵束 superior longitudinal band
2. 舌下神经管 hypoglossal canal
3. 翼状韧带 alar ligament
4. 后纵韧带 posterior longitudinal liga-
　ment
5. 寰枢外侧关节 lateral atlantoaxial joint
6. 寰椎横韧带 transverse ligament of atlas
7. 寰枕关节 atlantooccipital joint
8. 齿突尖韧带 apical ligament of dens
9. 覆膜 membrana tectoria
10. 颈内动脉 internal carotid artery
11. 内耳门 internal acoustic pore
12. 颈静脉孔 jugular foramen
13. 枢椎齿突 dens of axis
14. 椎动脉 vertebral artery
15. 下纵束 inferior longitudinal band
16. 外耳门 external acoustic pore
17. 颞骨茎突 styloid process of temporal
　bone
18. 颞骨乳突 mastoid process of temporal
　bone
19. 关节突关节 zygapophysial joints
20. 项韧带 ligamentum nuchae

B

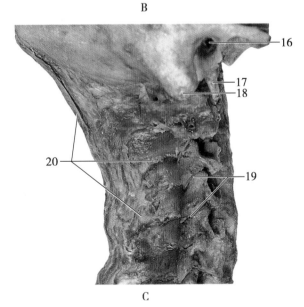

C

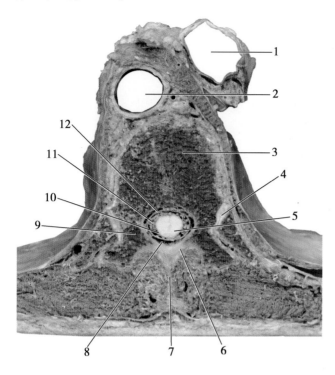

图7-11 椎管(胸段,上面观)
Vertebral canal(in thoracic region, superior view)

1. 下腔静脉 inferior vena cava
2. 胸主动脉 thoracic aorta
3. 椎体 vertebral body
4. 关节突关节 zygapophysial joint
5. 脊髓 spinal cord
6. 椎弓板 lamina of vertebral arch
7. 棘间韧带 interspinous ligament
8. 硬膜外隙 epidural space
9. 椎弓根 pedicle of vertebral arch
10. 蛛网膜(贴脊髓外表面) arachnoid mater(covers spinal cord)
11. 脊神经根 nerve roots
12. 硬脊膜 spinal dura mater

图7-12 椎间孔(右侧面观)
Intervertebral foramen(right lateral view)

1. 前纵韧带 anterior longitudinal ligament
2. 髓核 nucleus pulposus
3. 椎体 vertebral body
4. 纤维环 anulus fibrosus
5. 后纵韧带 posterior longitudinal ligament
6. 椎间盘 intervertebral disc
7. 上关节突 superior articular process
8. 黄韧带 ligamentum flavum
9. 椎弓板 lamina of vertebral arch
10. 椎弓根 pedicle of vertebral arch
11. 黄韧带 ligamentum flavum
12. 椎间孔 intervertebral foramen

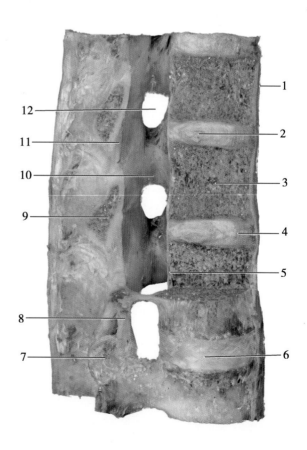

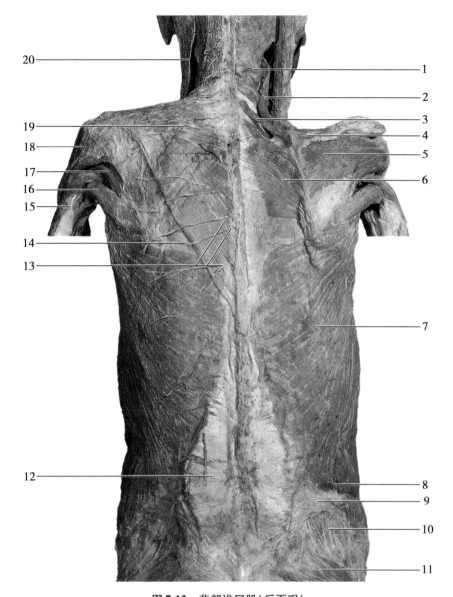

图 7-13 背部浅层肌（后面观）
Superficial muscles of back（posterior view）

1. 头夹肌 splenius capitis
2. 肩胛提肌 levator scapulae
3. 小菱形肌 rhomboideus minor
4. 冈上肌 supraspinatus
5. 冈下肌 infraspinatus
6. 大菱形肌 rhomboideus major
7. 背阔肌 latissimus dorsi
8. 腰下三角 inferior lumbar triangle
9. 髂嵴 iliac crest
10. 臀中肌 gluteus medius
11. 臀大肌 gluteus maximus
12. 胸腰筋膜 thoracolumbar fascia
13. 胸神经后支 dorsal ramus of thoracic nerve
14. 听诊三角 triangle of auscultation
15. 肱三头肌 triceps brachii
16. 大圆肌 teres major
17. 小圆肌 teres minor
18. 三角肌 deltoid
19. 斜方肌 trapezius
20. 胸锁乳突肌 sternocleidomastoid

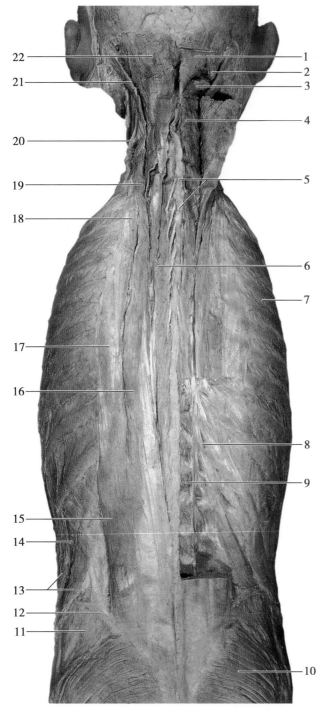

图 7-14 背部深层肌（后面观）
Deep muscles of back
（posterior view）

1. 头后大直肌 rectus capitis posterior major
2. 头上斜肌 obliquus capitis superior
3. 头下斜肌 obliquus capitis inferior
4. 颈半棘肌 semispinalis cervicis
5. 棘间肌 interspinales
6. 棘肌 spinalis
7. 肋间外肌 external intercostal
8. 肋提肌 levatores costarum
9. 横突间肌 intertransversarii
10. 臀大肌 gluteus maximus
11. 臀中肌 gluteus medius
12. 髂嵴 iliac crest
13. 腹外斜肌 obliquus externus abdominis
14. 腹内斜肌 obliquus internus abdominis
15. 腰髂肋肌 iliocostalis lumborum
16. 胸最长肌 longissimus thoracis
17. 胸髂肋肌 iliocostalis thoracis
18. 颈髂肋肌 iliocostalis cervicis
19. 颈最长肌 longissimus cervicis
20. 后斜角肌 scalenus posterior
21. 头最长肌 longissimus capitis
22. 头半棘肌 semispinalis capitis

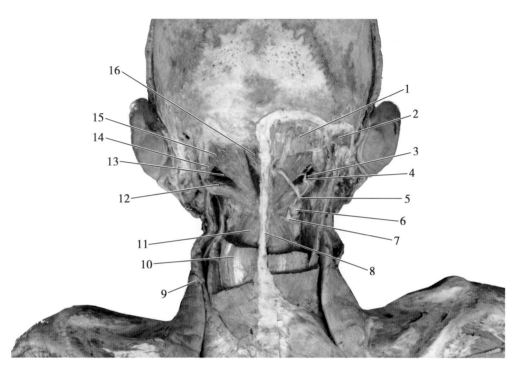

图 7-15　枕下三角(后面观)
Suboccipital triangle(posterior view)

1. 头半棘肌 semispinalis capitis
2. 头夹肌 splenius capitis
3. 椎动脉 vertebral artery
4. 第一颈脊神经后支(枕下神经)dorsal ramus of first cervical nerve(suboccipital nerve)
5. 第二颈脊神经后支(枕大神经) dorsal ramus of second cervical nerve(greater occipital nerve)
6. 枢椎横突 transverse process of axis
7. 第三颈神经后支(第三枕神经)dorsal ramus of third cervical nerve(third occipital nerve)
8. 项韧带 ligamentum nuchae
9. 肩胛提肌 levator scapulae
10. 头半棘肌 semispinalis capitis
11. 颈半棘肌 semispinalis cervicis
12. 头下斜肌 obliquus capitis inferior
13. 椎动脉 vertebral artery
14. 头上斜肌 obliquus capitis superior
15. 头后大直肌 rectus capitis posterior major
16. 头后小直肌 rectus capitis posterior minor

第 8 章 头与颈

Chapter 8　Head and Neck

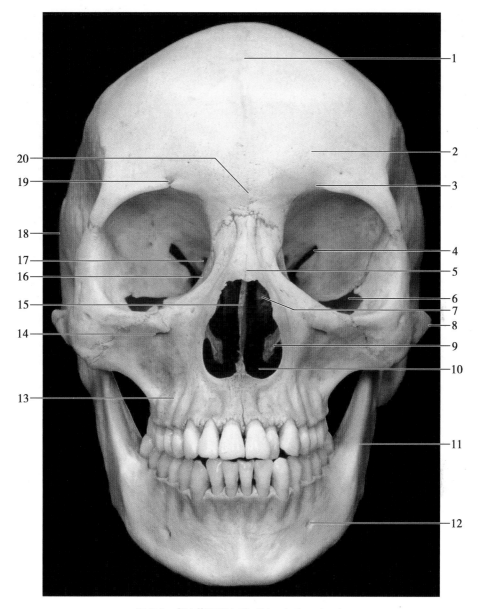

图 8-1　颅（前面观）Skull（anterior view）

1. 额骨 frontal bone
2. 眉弓 superciliary arch
3. 眶上切迹 supraorbital notch
4. 眶上裂 superior orbital fissure
5. 鼻骨 nasal bone
6. 眶下裂 inferior orbital fissure
7. 中鼻甲 middle nasal concha
8. 颧骨 zygomatic bone
9. 下鼻甲 inferior nasal concha
10. 梨状孔 piriform aperture
11. 下颌支 ramus of mandible
12. 颏孔 mental foramen
13. 上颌骨 maxilla
14. 眶下孔 infraorbital foramen
15. 鼻中隔 nasal septum
16. 泪骨 lacrimal bone
17. 视神经管 optic canal
18. 颞骨 temporal bone
19. 眶上孔 supraorbital foramen
20. 眉间 glabella

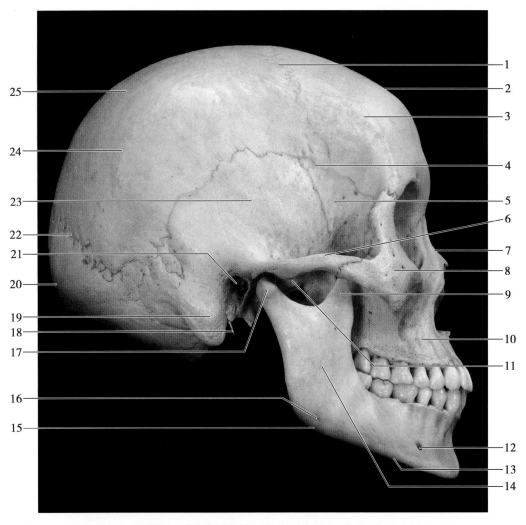

图 8-2 颅(右侧面观) Skull(right lateral view)

1. 冠状缝 coronal suture
2. 额骨 frontal bone
3. 上颞线 superior temporal line
4. 翼点 pterion
5. 蝶骨大翼 greater wing of sphenoid bone
6. 颞骨颧突 zygomatic process of temporal bone
7. 鼻骨 nasal bone
8. 颧骨 zygomatic bone
9. 下颌骨冠突 coronoid process of mandible
10. 上颌骨 maxilla
11. 关节结节 articular tubercle
12. 颏孔 mental foramen
13. 下颌体 body of mandible

14. 下颌支 ramus of mandible
15. 下颌角 angle of mandible
16. 咬肌粗隆 masseteric tuberosity
17. 下颌骨髁突 condylar process of mandible
18. 颞骨茎突 styloid process of temporal bone
19. 颞骨乳突 mastoid process of temporal bone
20. 枕骨 occipital bone
21. 外耳门 external acoustic meatus
22. 人字缝 lambdoid suture
23. 颞骨 temporal bone
24. 下颞线 inferior temporal line
25. 顶骨 parietal bone

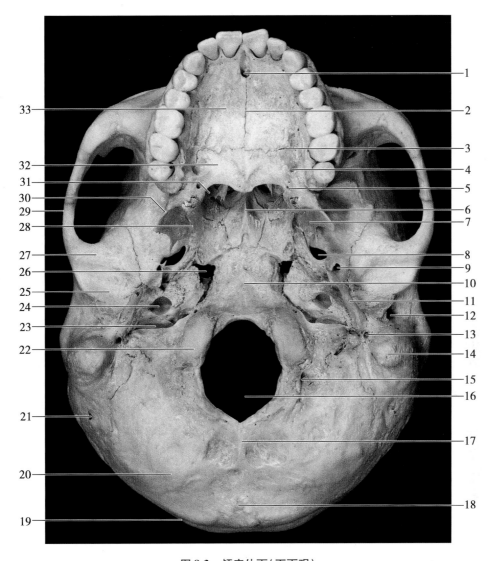

图 8-3 颅底外面(下面观)
External surface of base of skull(inferior view)

1. 切牙孔 incisive fossa
2. 腭正中缝 median palatine suture
3. 腭横缝 transverse palatine suture
4. 腭大孔 greater palatine foramen
5. 腭小孔 lesser palatine foramen
6. 犁骨 vomer
7. 翼窝 pterygoid fossa
8. 卵圆孔 foramen ovale
9. 棘孔 foramen spinosum
10. 咽结节 pharyngeal tubercle
11. 颞骨茎突 styloid process of temporal bone
12. 外耳门 external acoustic meatus
13. 茎乳孔 stylomastoid foramen
14. 颞骨乳突 mastoid process of temporal bone
15. 髁管 condylar canal
16. 枕骨大孔 foramen magnum
17. 枕外嵴 external occipital crest

18. 枕外隆凸 external occipital protuberance
19. 上项线 superior nuchal line
20. 下项线 inferior nuchal line
21. 乳突孔 mastoid foramen
22. 枕髁 occipital condyle
23. 颈静脉窝 jugular fossa
24. 颈动脉管外口 external aperture of carotid canal
25. 下颌窝 mandibular fossa
26. 破裂孔 foramen lacerum
27. 关节结节 articular tubercle
28. 翼突内侧板 medial pterygoid plate
29. 颧弓 zygomatic arch
30. 翼突外侧板 lateral pterygoid plate
31. 鼻后孔 posterior nasal aperture
32. 腭骨水平板 horizontal plate of palatine bone
33. 上颌骨腭突 palatine process of maxilla

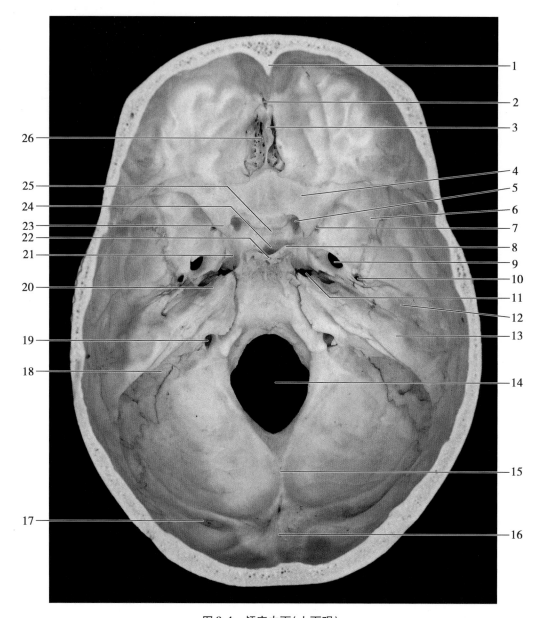

图 8-4 颅底内面(上面观)
Internal surface of base of skull (superior view)

1. 额嵴 frontal crest
2. 盲孔 foramen cecum
3. 鸡冠 crista galli
4. 蝶骨小翼 lesser wing of sphenoid bone
5. 视神经管 optic canal
6. 蝶骨大翼 greater wing of sphenoid bone
7. 圆孔 foramen rotundum
8. 后床突 posterior clinoid process
9. 卵圆孔 foramen ovale
10. 棘孔 foramen spinosum
11. 破裂孔 foramen lacerum
12. 鼓室盖 tegmen tympani
13. 弓状隆起 arcuate eminence
14. 枕骨大孔 foramen magnum
15. 枕内嵴 internal occipital crest
16. 枕内隆凸 internal occipital protuberance
17. 横窦沟 groove for transverse sinus
18. 乙状窦沟 groove for sigmoid sinus
19. 颈静脉孔 jugular foramen
20. 三叉神经压迹 trigeminal impression
21. 颈动脉沟 carotid sulcus
22. 鞍背 dorsum sellae
23. 前床突 anterior clinoid process
24. 垂体窝 hypophysial fossa
25. 交叉前沟 sulcus prechiasmaticus
26. 筛板 cribriform plate

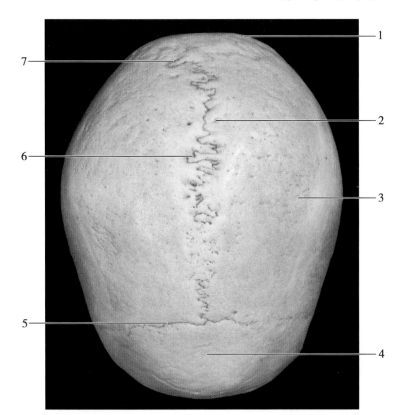

图 8-5 颅顶外面（上面观）
External surface of cranial vault（superior view）
1. 枕骨 occipital bone
2. 顶孔 parietal foramen
3. 顶骨 parietal bone
4. 额骨 frontal bone
5. 冠状缝 coronal suture
6. 矢状缝 sagittal suture
7. 人字缝 lambdoid suture

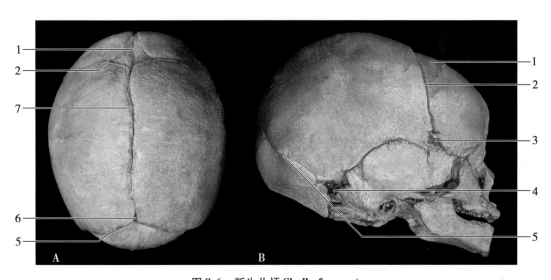

图 8-6 新生儿颅 Skull of neonate
A. 上面观 superior view　B. 右侧面观 right lateral view
1. 前囟 anterior fontanelle
2. 冠状缝 coronal suture
3. 前外侧（蝶）囟 anterolateral（sphenoidal）fontanelle
4. 后外侧（乳突）囟 posterolateral（mastoid）fontanelle
5. 人字缝 lambdoid suture
6. 后囟 posterior fontanelle
7. 矢状缝 sagittal suture

图 8-7　右眶(前面观)
Right orbit(anterior view)

1. 眶上切迹 supraorbital notch
2. 筛后孔 posterior ethmoidal foramen
3. 视神经管 optic canal
4. 筛骨眶板 orbital plate of ethmoid
5. 泪囊窝 fossa for lacrimal sac
6. 泪后嵴 posterior lacrimal crest
7. 上颌骨眶板 orbital plate of maxilla
8. 上颌骨 maxilla
9. 眶下孔 infraorbital foramen
10. 颧骨 zygomatic bone
11. 眶下沟 infraorbital groove
12. 眶下裂 inferior orbital fissure
13. 蝶骨眶面 orbital surface of sphenoid bone
14. 眶上裂 superior orbital fissure
15. 泪腺窝 fossa for lacrimal gland
16. 眶上缘 supraorbital margin

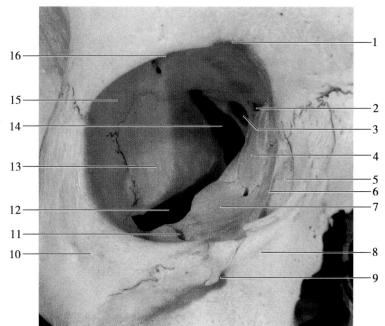

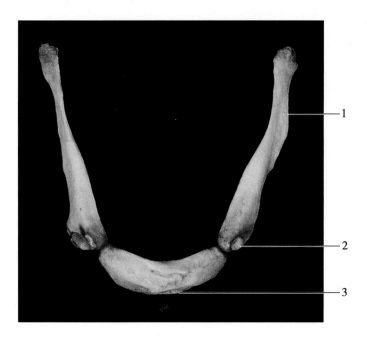

图 8-8　舌骨(上面观)
Hyoid bone(superior view)

1. 大角 greater cornu of hyoid bone
2. 小角 lesser cornu of hyoid bone
3. 舌骨体 body of hyoid bone

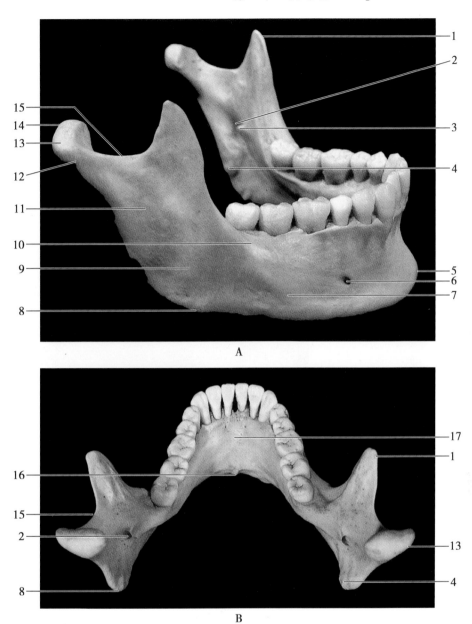

A

B

图 8-9 下颌骨 Mandible

A. 右外上面观 Right superolateral view B. 后上面观 Superoposterior view

1. 下颌骨冠突 coronoid process of mandible
2. 下颌孔 mandibular foramen
3. 下颌小舌 mandibular lingula
4. 翼肌粗隆 pterygoid tuberosity
5. 颏隆凸 mental protuberance
6. 颏孔 mental foramen
7. 下颌体 body of mandible
8. 下颌角 angle of mandible
9. 咬肌粗隆 masseteric tuberosity

10. 斜线 oblique line
11. 下颌支 ramus of mandible
12. 下颌颈 neck of mandible
13. 下颌头 head of mandible
14. 髁突 condylar process
15. 下颌切迹 mandibular notch
16. 颏棘 mental spine
17. 舌下腺凹 sublingual fossa

图 8-10 蝶骨 Sphenoid bone

A. 前面观 Anterior view
B. 后面观 Posterior view
C. 上面观 Superior view

1. 蝶骨小翼 lesser wing of sphenoid bone
2. 眶上裂 superior orbital fissure
3. 蝶骨大翼 greater wing of sphenoid bone
4. 蝶骨眶面 orbital surface of sphenoid bone
5. 圆孔 foramen rotundum
6. 翼管 pterygoid canal
7. 蝶棘 spine of sphenoid bone
8. 翼突内侧板 medial pterygoid plate
9. 翼突外侧板 lateral pterygoid plate
10. 蝶骨体 body of sphnoid bone
11. 蝶嵴 sphenoid crest
12. 蝶窦口 aperture of sphenoidal sinus
13. 蝶甲 sphenoidal concha
14. 视神经管 optic canal
15. 前床突 anterior clinoid process
16. 垂体窝 hypophysial fossa
17. 交叉前沟 sulcus prechiasmaticus
18. 卵圆孔 foramen ovale
19. 棘孔 foramen spinosum

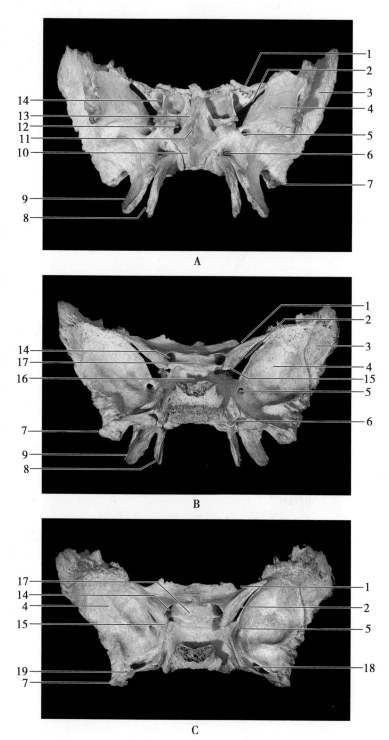

A

B

C

图 8-11 右颞骨 Right temporal bone

A. 外面观 External view

B. 内面观 Internal view

C. 下面观 Inferior view

1. 鳞部 squamous part
2. 颧突 zygomatic process
3. 关节结节 articular tubercle
4. 下颌窝 mandibular fossa
5. 鼓部 tympanic part
6. 茎突 styloid process
7. 鼓乳裂 tympanomastoid fissure
8. 乳突 mammillary process
9. 道上嵴 suprameatal spine
10. 道上三角 suprameatal triangle
11. 外耳道 external acoustic meatus
12. 鼓室盖 tegmen tympani
13. 弓状隆起 arcuate eminence
14. 三叉神经压迹 trigeminal impression
15. 前庭水管外口 external aperture of aqueduct of vestibule
16. 岩上窦沟 groove for superior petrosal sinus
17. 乙状窦沟 groove for sigmoid sinus
18. 颈动脉管 carotid canal
19. 颈静脉窝 jugular fossa
20. 茎乳孔 stylomastoid foramen
21. 枕动脉沟 occipital groove
22. 乳突切迹 mastoid notch
23. 岩鼓裂 petrotympanic fissure
24. 岩鳞裂 petrosquamous fissure
25. 肌咽鼓管 musculotubal canal

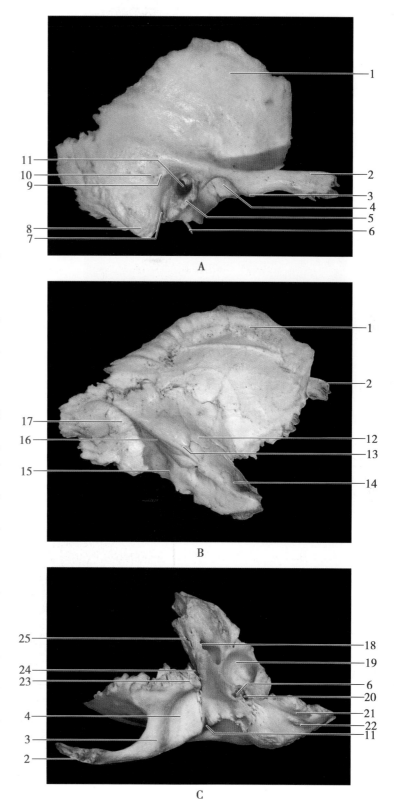

A

B

C

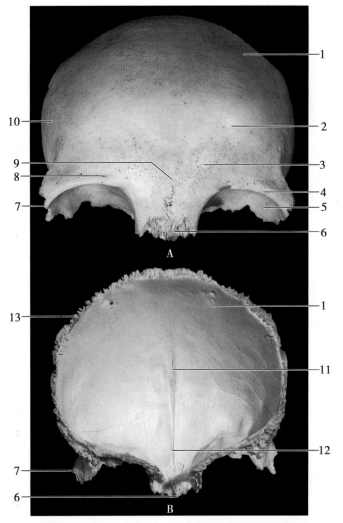

图 8-12　额骨 **Frontal bone**
　A. 前面观 Anterior view
　B. 后面观 Posterior view
1. 额鳞 frontal squama
2. 额结节 frontal eminence
3. 眉弓 superciliary arch
4. 泪腺窝 fossa for lacrimal gland
5. 眶上缘 supraorbital margin
6. 鼻缘 nasal margin
7. 颧突 zygomatic process
8. 眶上孔 supraorbital foramen
9. 眉间 glabella
10. 颞线 temporal line
11. 上矢状窦沟 groove for superior sagittal sinus
12. 额嵴 frontal crest
13. 顶缘 parietal margin

图 8-13　筛骨 **Ethmoid**
　A. 上面观 Superior view
　B. 下面观 Inferior view
1. 垂直板 perpendicular plate
2. 筛骨迷路 ethmoidal labyrinth
3. 中鼻甲 middle nasal concha
4. 上鼻甲 superior nasal concha
5. 眶板 orbital plate
6. 筛孔 foramina of cribriform plate
7. 筛板 cribriform plate
8. 鸡冠 crista galli

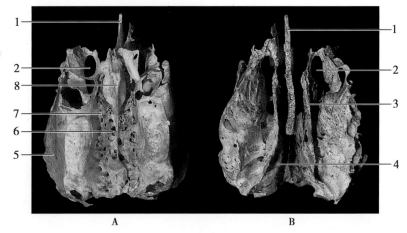

图 8-14 枕骨 Occipital bone

A. 外面观 External view

B. 内面观 Internal view

1. 枕鳞 occipital squama
2. 枕外隆凸 external occipital protuberance
3. 枕外嵴 external occipital crest
4. 髁管 condylar canal
5. 枕髁 occipital condyle
6. 咽结节 pharyngeal tubercle
7. 枕骨大孔 foramen magnum
8. 下项线 inferior nuchal line
9. 上项线 superior nuchal line
10. 最上项线 highest nuchal line
11. 大脑窝 cerebral fossa
12. 枕内隆凸 internal occipital protuberance
13. 枕内嵴 internal occipital crest
14. 小脑窝 cerebellar fossa
15. 基底部 basilar part
16. 横窦沟 groove for transverse sinus
17. 上矢状窦沟 groove for superior sagittal sinus

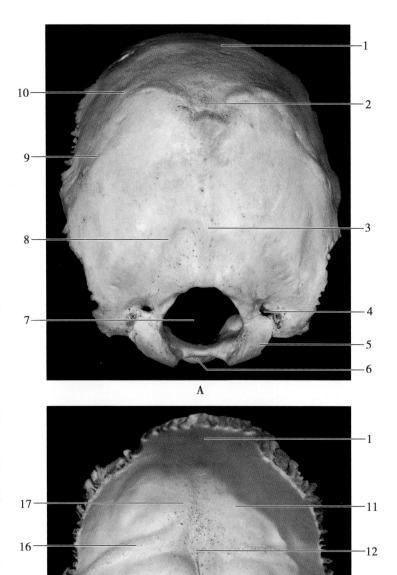

A

B

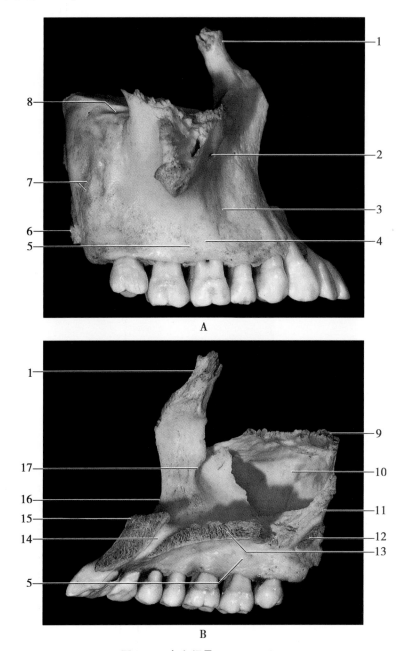

A

B

图 8-15　右上颌骨 Right maxilla
A. 外面观 Lateral view
B. 内面观 Medial view

1. 额突 frontal process
2. 眶下孔 infraorbital foramen
3. 尖牙窝 canine fossa
4. 牙槽轭 juga alveolaria
5. 牙槽突 alveolar process
6. 上颌结节 tuberosity of maxilla
7. 牙槽孔 alveolar foramina
8. 眶下裂 inferior orbital fissure
9. 颧突 zygomatic process
10. 上颌窦裂孔 maxillary hiatus
11. 腭大沟 greater palatine groove
12. 腭小沟 lesser palatine groove
13. 腭突 palatine process
14. 切牙管 incisive canal
15. 鼻前棘 anterior nasal spine
16. 鼻切迹 nasal notch
17. 泪沟 lacrimal groove

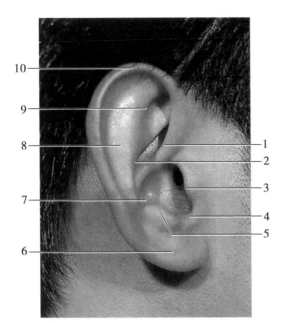

图 8-16 右耳廓 Right auricle

1. 耳轮脚 crus of helix
2. 对耳轮脚 crura of antihelix
3. 耳屏 tragus
4. 耳屏间切迹 intertragic notch
5. 对耳屏 antitragus
6. 耳垂 auricular lobule
7. 耳甲 concha of auricle
8. 耳舟 scapha
9. 对耳轮 antihelix
10. 耳轮 helix

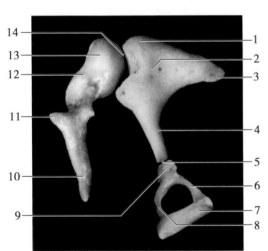

图 8-17 听小骨 Auditory ossicles

1. 砧骨 incus
2. 砧骨体 body of incus
3. 砧骨短脚 short limb of incus
4. 砧骨长脚 long limb of incus
5. 砧镫关节 incudostapedial joint
6. 镫骨后脚 posterior process of stapes
7. 镫骨底 base of stapes
8. 镫骨前脚 anterior process of stapes
9. 镫骨 stapes
10. 锤骨柄 handle of malleus
11. 锤骨前突 anterior process of malleus
12. 锤骨颈 neck of malleus
13. 锤骨头 head of malleus
14. 砧锤关节 incudomalleolar joint

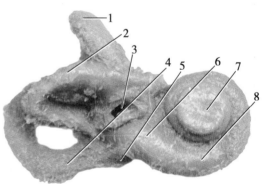

图 8-18 骨迷路 Bony labyrinth

1. 前半规管 anterior semicircular canal
2. 外半规管 lateral semicircular canal
3. 前庭窗(卵圆窗) fenestra vestibule(oval window)
4. 后半规管 posterior semicircular canal
5. 蜗窗(圆窗) fenestra cochleae(round window)
6. 前庭 vestibule
7. 蜗顶 cupula of cochlea
8. 耳蜗 cochlea

175

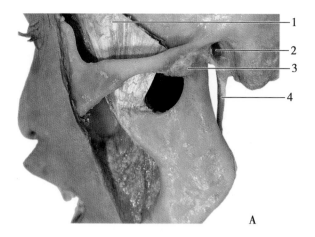

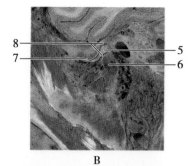

B

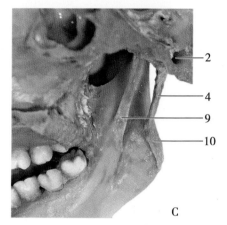

C

图 8-19　左颞下颌关节 Left temporomandibular joint

　　　　A. 外面观 Lateral view
　　　　B. 矢状剖面 Sagittal section of joint
　　　　C. 前外面观 Anterolateral view

1. 颞肌 temporalis
2. 外耳道 external acoustic meatus
3. 关节囊 articular capsule
4. 颞骨茎突 styloid process of temporal bone
5. 关节盘 articular disc
6. 髁突 condylar process
7. 关节结节 articular tubercle
8. 关节腔 articular cavities
9. 蝶下颌韧带 sphenomandibular ligament
10. 茎突下颌韧带 stylomandibular ligament

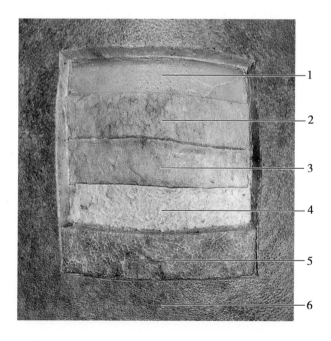

图 8-20　头皮 Scalp

1. 颅顶 cranial vault
2. 颅骨膜 pericranium
3. 帽状腱膜下间隙 subaponeurotic space
4. 帽状腱膜 galea aponeurotica
5. 皮下组织 subcutaneous tissue
6. 皮肤 skin

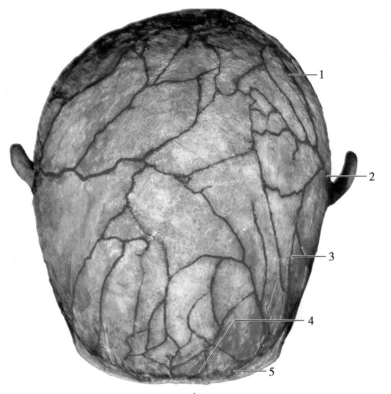

图 8-21 头皮的血管（上面观）
Blood vessels of scalp
（superior view）
  A. 动脉 Arteries
  B. 静脉 Veins
1. 枕动脉 occipital artery
2. 耳后动脉 posterior auricular artery
3. 颞浅动脉 superficial temporal artery
4. 滑车动脉 supratrochlear artery
5. 眶上动脉 supraorbital artery

1. 滑车静脉 supratrochlear vein
2. 眶上静脉 supraorbital vein
3. 颞浅静脉 superficial temporal vein
4. 耳后静脉 posterior auricular vein
5. 枕静脉 occipital vein

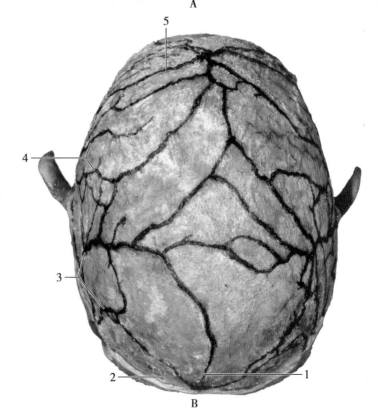

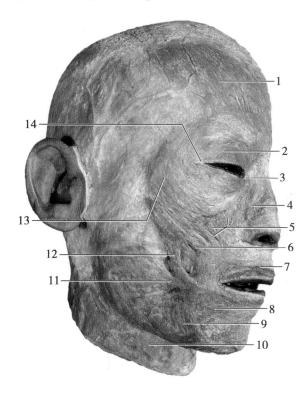

图 8-22　表情肌（右前外侧面观）
Muscles of facial expresion（right anterolateral view）

1. 枕额肌额腹 frontal belly of occipitofrontalis
2. 眼轮匝肌睑部 palpebral part of orbicularis oculi
3. 睑内侧韧带 medial palpebral ligament
4. 提上唇鼻翼肌 levator labii superioris alaeque nasi
5. 提上唇肌 levator labii superioris
6. 颧小肌 zygomaticus minor
7. 口轮匝肌 orbicularis oris
8. 降下唇肌 depressor labii inferioris
9. 降口角肌 depressor anguli oris
10. 颈阔肌 platysma
11. 笑肌 risorius
12. 颧大肌 zygomaticus major
13. 眼轮匝肌眶部 orbital part of orbicularis oculi
14. 睑外侧韧带 lateral palpebral ligament

图 8-23　头颈浅结构（右外侧面观）
Superficial structures of head and neck（right lateral view）

1. 耳颞神经 auriculotemporal nerve
2. 颞浅动脉和静脉 superficial temporal artery and vein
3. 眼轮匝肌 orbicularis oculi
4. 面神经（Ⅶ）颞支 temporal branches of facial nerve（Ⅶ）
5. 面神经（Ⅶ）颧支 zygomatic branches of facial nerve（Ⅶ）
6. 副腮腺 accessory parotid gland
7. 腮腺管 parotid duct
8. 面神经（Ⅶ）颊支 buccal branches of facial nerve（Ⅶ）
9. 面动脉 facial artery
10. 面神经（Ⅶ）下颌缘支 marginal mandibular branches of facial nerve（Ⅶ）
11. 面神经（Ⅶ）颈支 cervical branches of facial nerve（Ⅶ）
12. 颈阔肌 platysma
13. 副神经（Ⅺ）accessory nerve（Ⅺ）
14. 耳大神经 great auricular nerve
15. 胸锁乳突肌 sternocleidomastoid
16. 枕小神经 lesser occipital nerve
17. 腮腺 parotid gland
18. 枕大神经和枕动脉 greater occipital nerve and occipital artery

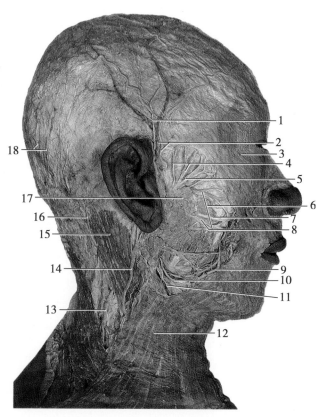

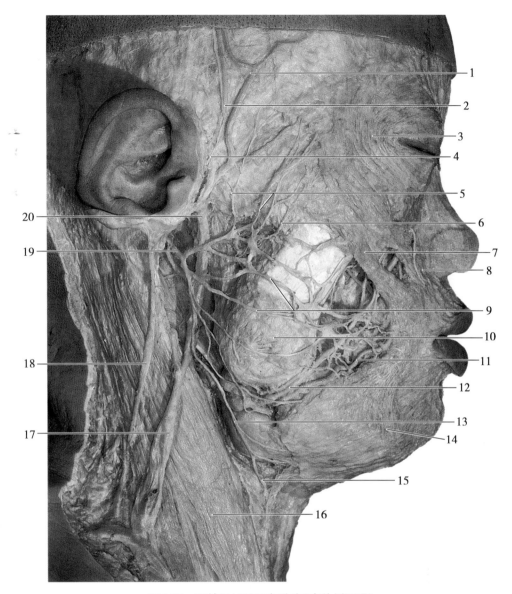

图 8-24 面神经(Ⅶ)面部分支(右外侧面观)
Branches of facial nerve(Ⅶ) on face(right lateral view)

1. 颞浅动脉 superficial temporal artery
2. 颞浅静脉 superficial temporal vein
3. 眼轮匝肌 orbicularis oculi
4. 耳颞神经 auriculotemporal nerve
5. 面神经(Ⅶ)颞支 temporal branches of facial nerve(Ⅶ)
6. 面神经(Ⅶ)颧支 zygomatic branches of facial nerve(Ⅶ)
7. 颧大肌 zygomaticus major
8. 提上唇肌 levator labii superioris
9. 面神经(Ⅶ)颊支 buccal branches of facial nerve(Ⅶ)
10. 咬肌 masseter
11. 面动脉 facial artery
12. 面静脉 facial vein
13. 面神经(Ⅶ)下颌缘支 marginal mandibular branches of facial nerve(Ⅶ)
14. 降口角肌 depressor anguli oris
15. 面神经(Ⅶ)颈支 cervical branches of facial nerve(Ⅶ)
16. 胸锁乳突肌 sternocleidomastoid
17. 颈外静脉 external jugular vein
18. 耳大神经 great auricular nerve
19. 面神经(Ⅶ) facial nerve(Ⅶ)
20. 下颌后静脉 retromandibular vein

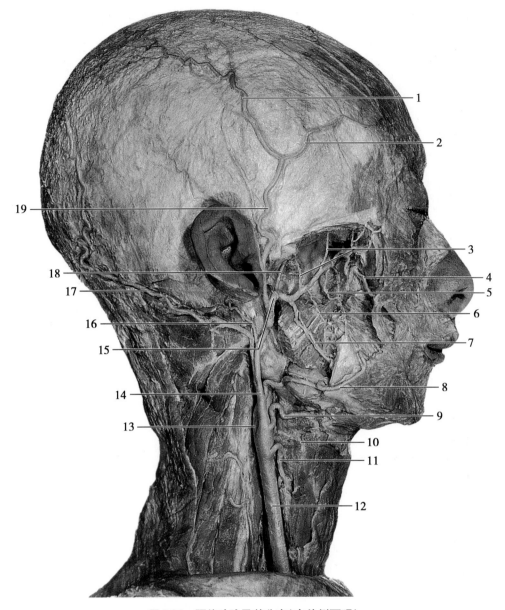

图 8-25 颈外动脉及其分支（右外侧面观）
External carotid artery and its branches (right lateral view)

1. 颞浅动脉顶支 parietal branch of superficial temporal artery
2. 颞浅动脉额支 frontal branch of superficial temporal artery
3. 颞深前、后动脉 anterior and posterior deep temporal arteries
4. 上牙槽后动脉 posterior superior alveolar artery
5. 颊动脉 buccal artery
6. 上颌动脉翼肌支 pterygoid branches of maxillary artery
7. 下牙槽动脉 inferior alveolar artery
8. 面动脉 facial artery
9. 舌动脉 lingual artery
10. 喉上动脉 superior laryngeal artery
11. 甲状腺上动脉 superior thyroid artery
12. 颈总动脉 common carotid artery
13. 颈内动脉 internal carotid artery
14. 颈外动脉 external carotid artery
15. 上颌动脉 maxillary artery
16. 耳后动脉 posterior auricular artery
17. 枕动脉 occipital artery
18. 脑膜中动脉 middle meningeal artery
19. 颞浅动脉 superficial temporal artery

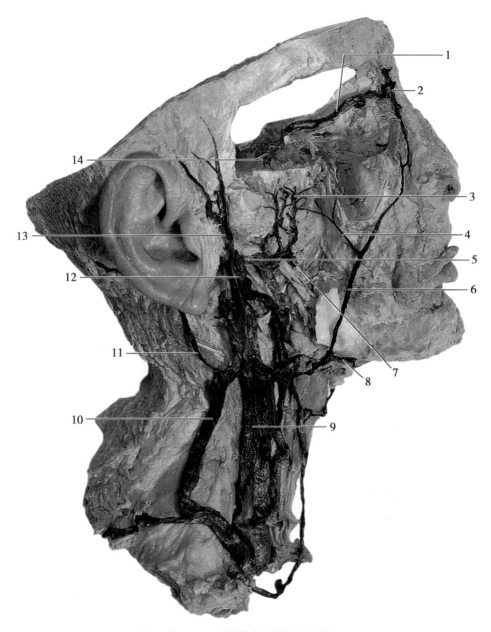

图 8-26　头颈静脉（右外侧面观）
Veins of head and neck（right lateral view）

1. 眼上静脉 superior ophthalmic vein
2. 内眦静脉 angular vein
3. 翼静脉丛 pterygoid venous plexus
4. 面深静脉 deep facial vein
5. 上颌静脉 maxillary vein
6. 面静脉 facial vein
7. 下牙槽静脉 inferior alveolar vein
8. 颏下静脉 submental vein
9. 颈内静脉 internal jugular vein
10. 颈外静脉 external jugular vein
11. 耳后静脉 posterior auricular vein
12. 下颌后静脉 retromandibular vein
13. 颞浅静脉 superficial temporal vein
14. 海绵窦 cavernous sinus

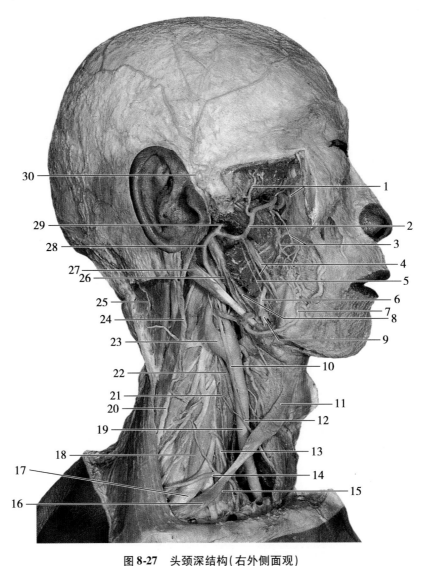

图 8-27 头颈深结构（右外侧面观）
Deep structures of head and neck（right lateral view）

1. 颞深前、后动脉 anterior and posterior deep temporal arteries
2. 上颌动脉 maxillary artery
3. 颊动脉和神经 buccal artery and nerve
4. 下牙槽神经和动脉 inferior alveolar nerve and artery
5. 下颌舌骨肌神经 nerve to mylohyoid
6. 舌神经 lingual nerve
7. 面动脉 facial artery
8. 茎突舌肌 styloglossus
9. 下颌下神经节 submandibular ganglion
10. 颈襻上根 superior root of ansa cervicalis
11. 肩胛舌骨肌上腹 superior belly of omohyoid
12. 颈襻 ansa cervicalis
13. 膈神经 phrenic nerve
14. 颈横动脉 transverse cervical artery
15. 前斜角肌 scalenus anterior
16. 肩胛舌骨肌下腹 inferior belly of omohyoid
17. 臂丛 brachial plexus
18. 中斜角肌 scaleuns medius
19. 颈总动脉 common carotid artery
20. 副神经（XI）accessory nerve（XI）
21. 颈襻下根 inferior root of ansa cervicalis
22. 迷走神经（X）vagus nerve（X）
23. 颈动脉窦 carotid sinus
24. 耳大神经 great auricular nerve
25. 枕小神经 lesser occipital nerve
26. 茎突舌骨肌 stylohyoid
27. 二腹肌后腹 posterior belly of digastric
28. 颈外动脉 external carotid artery
29. 脑膜中动脉 middle meningeal artery
30. 颞浅动脉 superficial temporal artery

182

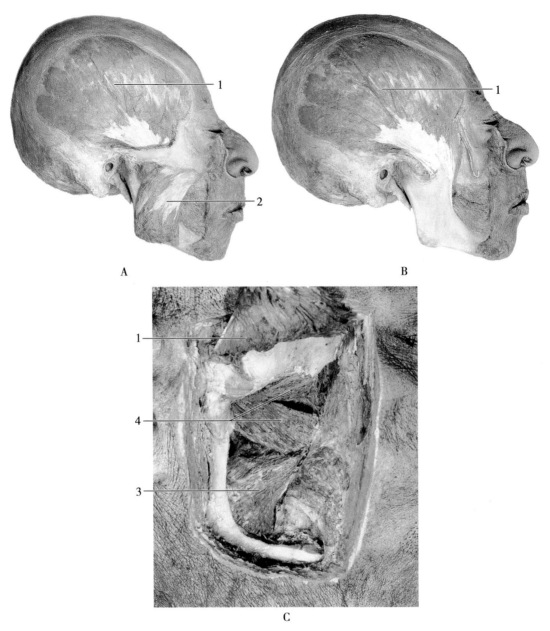

图 8-28　咀嚼肌(右外侧面观)
Muscles of mastication (right lateral view)
A. 咬肌和颞肌 Masseter and temporalis
B. 颧弓已移除 Zygomatic arch has been removed
C. 下颌骨支和体大部已移除 Most of ramus and body of mandible have been removed

1. 颞肌 temporalis
2. 咬肌 masseter
3. 翼内肌 medial pterygoid
4. 翼外肌 lateral pterygoid

1. 翼腭神经节 pterygopalatine ganglion
2. 眼神经 ophthalmic nerve
3. 上颌神经 maxillary nerve
4. 三叉神经（Ⅴ）trigeminal nerve（Ⅴ）
5. 颈内动脉 internal carotid artery
6. 三叉神经节 trigeminal ganglion
7. 下颌神经 mandibular nerve
8. 鼓索 chorda tympanic
9. 面神经（Ⅶ）facial nerve（Ⅶ）
10. 上颌动脉 maxillary artery
11. 下牙槽神经 inferior alveolar nerve
12. 翼内肌 medial pterygoid
13. 下牙槽动脉下颌舌骨肌支 mylohyoid branch of inferior alveolar artery
14. 下牙槽神经下颌舌骨肌支 mylohyoid branch of inferior alveolar nerve
15. 二腹肌前腹 anterior belly of digastric

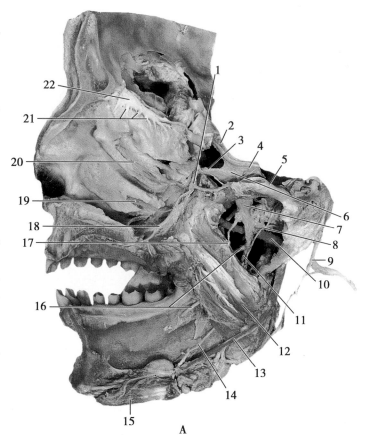

A

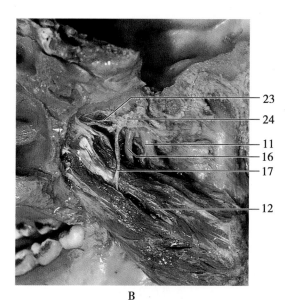

B

16. 舌神经 lingual nerve
17. 下颌神经翼内肌支 medial pterygoid branch of mandibular nerve
18. 腭大神经 greater palatine nerve
19. 下后外侧鼻神经 posterior inferior lateral nasal nerve
20. 上后外侧鼻神经 posterior superior lateral nasal nerve
21. 嗅神经（Ⅰ）olfactory nerve（Ⅰ）
22. 嗅球 olfactory bulb
23. 岩大神经 greater petrosal nerve
24. 耳神经节 otic ganglion

图 8-29　三叉神经（Ⅴ）Trigeminal nerve（Ⅴ）
A. 右内侧面观 Right medial view　B. 耳节 Otic ganglion

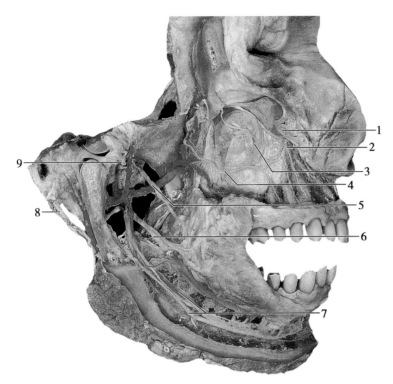

图 8-30 三叉神经(V)(右
外侧面观)
**Trigeminal nerve(V)(right
lateral view)**
1. 眶下神经 infraorbital nerve
2. 上牙槽前神经 anterior supe-
rior alveolar nerve
3. 上牙槽中神经 middle superi-
or alveolar nerve
4. 上牙槽后神经 posterior su-
perior alveolar nerve
5. 颊神经 buccal nerve
6. 舌神经 lingual nerve
7. 下牙槽神经和动脉 inferior
alveolar nerve and artery
8. 面神经(Ⅶ) facial nerve(Ⅶ)
9. 下颌神经 mandibular nerve

1. 泪腺 lacrimal gland
2. 上颌神经 maxillary nerve
3. 翼腭神经节 pterygopalatine ganglion
4. 鼻腭黏膜腺 nasal and palatal glands
5. 耳神经节 otic ganglion
6. 腮腺 parotid gland
7. 下颌神经 mandibular nerve
8. 舌神经 lingual nerve
9. 舌 tongue
10. 下颌下神经节 submandibular ganglion
11. 舌下腺 sublingual gland
12. 下颌下腺 submandibular gland
13. 耳颞神经 auriculotemporal nerve
14. 舌咽神经(Ⅸ) glossopharyngeal nerve
(Ⅸ)
15. 面神经(Ⅶ) facial nerve(Ⅶ)
16. 鼓索 chorda tympanic
17. 鼓室丛 tympanic plexus
18. 膝神经节 geniculate ganglion
19. 孤束核 nucleus of solitary tract
20. 孤束 solitary tract
21. 面神经核 facial motor nucleus
22. 上泌涎核 superior salivatory nucleus
23. 岩大神经 greater petrosal nerve
24. 岩小神经 lesser petrosal nerve

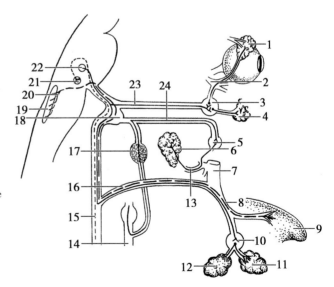

图 8-31 面神经(Ⅶ)和舌咽神经(Ⅸ)的副交感纤
维分布模式图
**Diagram for distribution of parasympathetic fibers
in facial and glossharyngeal nerve(Ⅶ and Ⅸ)**

185

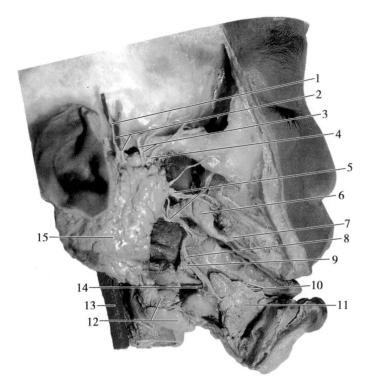

图 8-32　大唾液腺（右外侧面观）
Large salivary glands（right lateral view）

1. 耳颞神经 auriculotemporal nerve
2. 颞浅动脉和静脉 superficial temporal artery and vein
3. 面神经（Ⅶ）颞支 temporal branches of facial nerve（Ⅶ）
4. 面神经（Ⅶ）颧支 zygomatic branches of facial nerve（Ⅶ）
5. 面神经（Ⅶ）颊支 buccal branches of facial nerve（Ⅶ）
6. 副腮腺 accessory parotid gland
7. 腮腺管 parotid duct
8. 舌神经 lingual nerve
9. 下颌下神经节 submandibular ganglion
10. 舌下腺管 sublingual duct
11. 舌下腺 sublingual gland
12. 下颌下腺 submandibular gland
13. 颈总动脉 common carotid artery
14. 下颌下腺管 submandibular duct
15. 腮腺 parotid gland

1. 舌神经 lingual nerve
2. 下颌下神经节 submandibular ganglion
3. 舌 tongue
4. 舌下腺 sublingual gland
5. 舌下神经（Ⅻ）hypoglossal nerve（Ⅻ）
6. 颏舌骨肌 geniohyoid
7. 舌动脉 lingual artery
8. 甲状舌骨肌 thyrohyoid
9. 甲状软骨 thyroid cartilage
10. 颈总动脉 common carotid artery
11. 咽下缩肌 inferior pharyngeal constrictor
12. 舌静脉 lingual vein
13. 下颌下腺 submandibular gland

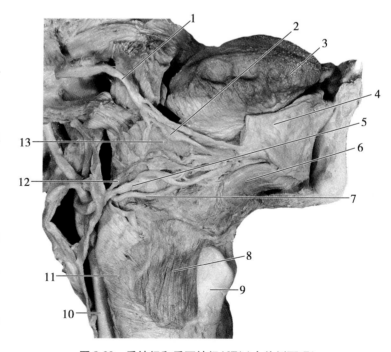

图 8-33　舌神经和舌下神经（Ⅻ）（右外侧面观）
Lingual nerve and hypoglossal nerve（Ⅻ）（right lateral view）

图 8-34 舌 Tongue

A. 背面 Dorsum

B. 矢状切面 Sagittal section

C. 冠状切面 Coronal section

1. 舌扁桃体 lingual tonsil

2. 轮廓乳头 vallate papillae

3. 叶状乳头 foliate papillae

4. 菌状乳头 fungiform papillae

5. 丝状乳头 filiform papillae

6. 舌尖 apex of tongue

7. 舌体 body of tongue

8. 舌根 root of tongue

1. 会厌 epiglottis

2. 舌上纵肌 superior longitudinal muscle of tongue

3. 舌垂直肌 vertical muscle of tongue

4. 舌骨 hyoid bone

5. 颏舌骨肌 geniohyoid

6. 颏舌肌 genioglossus

7. 舌下纵肌 inferior longitudinal muscle of tongue

8. 舌横肌 transverse muscle of tongue

9. 舌背 dorsum of tongue

10. 舌黏膜 lingual mucous membrane

11. 舌动脉 lingual artery

12. 舌中隔 septum of tongue

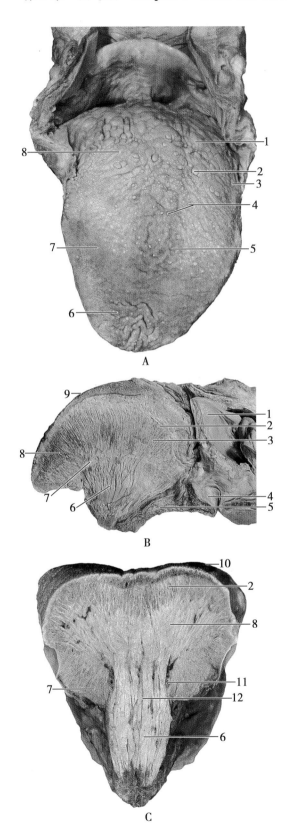

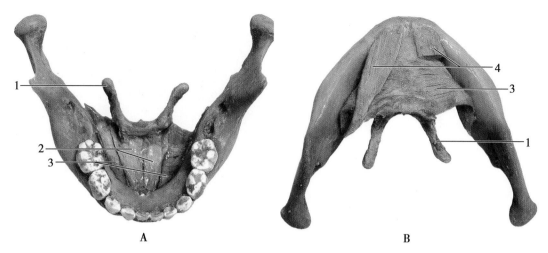

图 8-35　口腔底肌 Muscular floor of oral cavity
A. 上面观 Superior view　B. 下面观 Inferior view
　1. 舌骨 hyoid bone
　2. 颏舌骨肌 geniohyoid
　3. 下颌舌骨肌 mylohyoid
　4. 二腹肌前腹 anterior belly of digastric

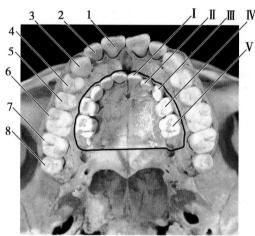

图 8-36　上颌恒、乳牙（下面观）
Upper permanent and deciduous
teeth（inferior view）
　1. 中切牙 central incisor
　2. 侧切牙 lateral incisor
　3. 尖牙 canine
　4. 第一前磨牙 first premolar
　5. 第二前磨牙 second premolar
　6. 第一磨牙 first molar
　7. 第二磨牙 second molar
　8. 第三磨牙 third molar

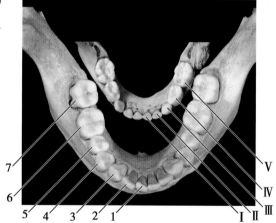

图 8-37　下颌恒、乳牙（上面观）
Lower permanent and deciduous
teeth（superior view）
　Ⅰ. 乳中切牙 deciduous central incisor
　Ⅱ. 乳侧切牙 deciduous lateral incisor
　Ⅲ. 尖牙 deciduous canine
　Ⅳ. 第一乳磨牙 first deciduous molar
　Ⅴ. 第二乳磨牙 second deciduous molar

188

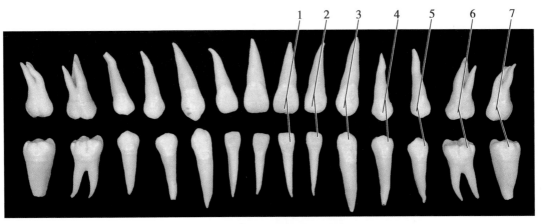

图 8-38　恒牙 **Permanent teeth**

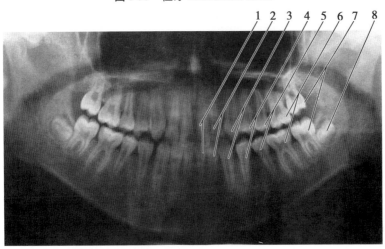

图 8-39　全颌曲面断层摄影 Orthopantomography of permanent teeth

1. 中切牙 central incisor
2. 侧切牙 lateral incisor
3. 尖牙 canine
4. 第一前磨牙 first premolar
5. 第二前磨牙 second premolar
6. 第一磨牙 first molar
7. 第二磨牙 second molar
8. 第三磨牙 third molar

9. 釉质 enamel
10. 牙本质 dentin
11. 牙髓 dental pulp
12. 牙骨质 cementum
13. 牙根管 root canal
14. 牙周膜 periodontium
15. 牙根尖孔 apical foramina
16. 牙槽骨 alveolar bone
17. 牙龈 gum
18. 牙腔 dental cavity

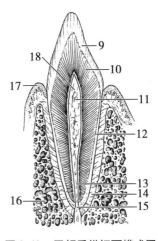

图 8-40　牙颊舌纵切面模式图
Diagram of a tooth sectioned in buccolingual longitudinal plane

189

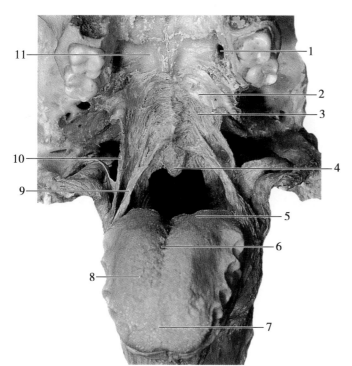

图 8-41 咽峡(前面观)
Pharyngeal isthmus(anterior view)
1. 腭大孔 greater palatine foramen
2. 腭帆张肌 tensor veli palatini
3. 软腭 soft palate
4. 腭垂 uvula
5. 舌根 root of tongue
6. 舌正中沟 median sulcus of tongue
7. 舌尖 apex of tongue
8. 舌体 body of tongue
9. 腭舌弓 palatoglossal arch
10. 腭咽弓 palatopharyngeal arch
11. 腭骨水平板 horizontal plate of palatine bone

1. 下鼻甲 inferior nasal concha
2. 腭帆张肌 tensor veli palatini
3. 软腭 soft palate
4. 茎突咽肌 stylopharyngeus
5. 茎突舌骨肌 stylohyoid
6. 腭咽肌 palatopharyngeus
7. 咽中缩肌 middle pharyngeal constrictor
8. 杓状会厌襞 aryepiglottic fold
9. 杓间切迹 interarytenoid notch
10. 咽下缩肌 inferior pharyngeal constrictor
11. 食管 esophagus
12. 梨状隐窝 piriform recess
13. 甲状软骨上角 superior cornu of thyroid cartilage
14. 会厌 epiglottis
15. 舌 tongue
16. 腭垂肌 musculus uvulae
17. 腭帆提肌 levator veli palatini
18. 鼻中隔 nasal septum

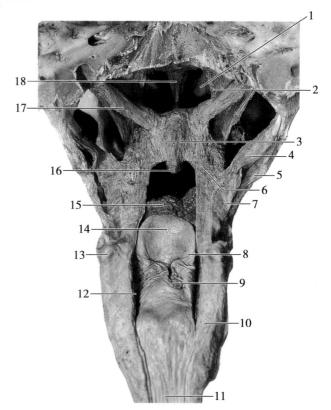

图 8-42 咽腔(后面观,咽后壁已被切开并推向两侧)
Pharyngeal cavity(posterior view, posterior wall of pharynx has been cut and reflected laterally on either side)

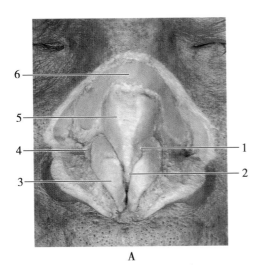
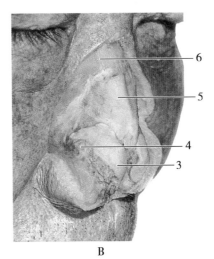

A　　　　　　　　　　　B

图 8-43　鼻的骨骼
Bony and cartilaginous skeleton of nose

A. 前面观 Anterior view　B. 右前外侧观 Right anterolateral view

1. 鼻副软骨 accessory nasal cartilages
2. 鼻隔软骨 septal cartilage
3. 鼻翼大软骨 major alar cartilage
4. 鼻翼小软骨 minor alar cartilages
5. 鼻隔软骨外侧突 lateral process of septal cartilage
6. 鼻骨 nasal bone

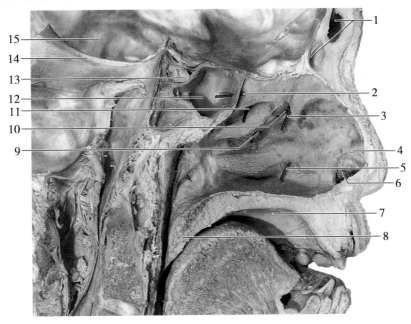

图 8-44　左侧鼻旁窦的开口(内侧面观)
Orifices of left paranasal sinuses(medial view)

1. 额窦 frontal sinus
2. 蝶窦开口 opening of sphenoidal sinus
3. 额窦开口 opening of frontal sinus
4. 鼻阈 nasal limen
5. 鼻泪管开口 opening of nasolacrimal duct
6. 鼻前庭 nasal vestibule
7. 硬腭 hard palate
8. 软腭 soft palate
9. 上颌窦开口 opening of maxillary sinus
10. 筛窦前群开口 opening of anterior ethmoidal cells
11. 筛窦后群开口 opening of posterior ethmoidal cells
12. 蝶窦 sphenoidal sinus
13. 垂体 pituitary gland
14. 小脑幕 tentorium of cerebellum
15. 硬脑膜 cerebral dura mater

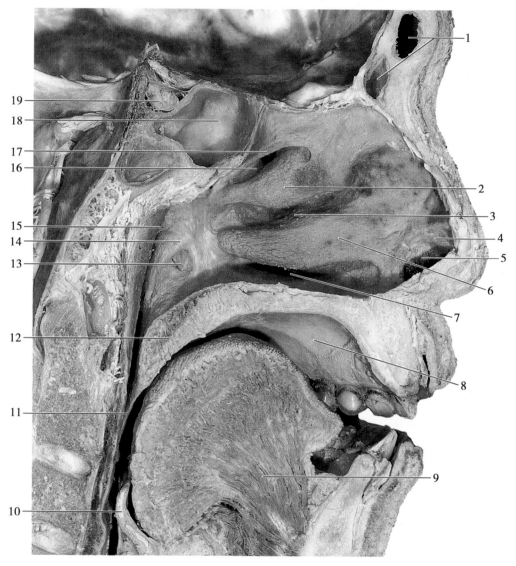

图 8-45 鼻腔左外侧壁 Left lateral wall of nasal cavity

1. 额窦 frontal sinus
2. 中鼻甲 middle nasal concha
3. 中鼻道 middle nasal meatus
4. 鼻阈 nasal limen
5. 鼻前庭 nasal vestibule
6. 下鼻甲 inferior nasal concha
7. 下鼻道 inferior nasal meatus
8. 硬腭 hard palate
9. 颏舌肌 genioglossus
10. 会厌 epiglottis
11. 腭咽弓 palatopharyngeal arch
12. 软腭 soft palate
13. 咽鼓管咽口 ostium of pharyngotympanic tube
14. 咽鼓管圆枕 tubal torus of pharyngotympanic tube
15. 咽隐窝 pharyngeal recess
16. 上鼻道 superior nasal meatus
17. 上鼻甲 superior nasal concha
18. 蝶窦 sphenoidal sinus
19. 垂体 pituitary gland

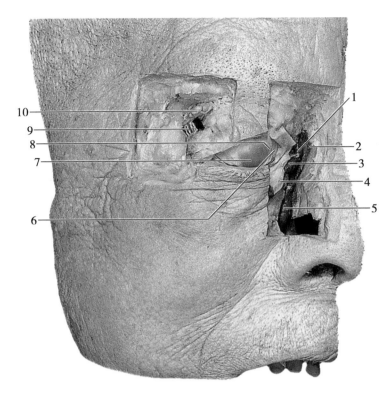

图 8-46 右泪器(前面观)
Right lacrimal apparatus
(anterior view)

1. 上泪小管 upper lacrimal canaliculus
2. 泪囊 lacrimal sac
3. 下泪小管 lower lacrimal canaliculus
4. 下泪点 inferior lacrimal puncta
5. 鼻泪管 nasolacrimal duct
6. 泪湖 lacrimal lake
7. 角膜 cornea
8. 结膜半月襞 conjunctival semilunar fold
9. 泪腺小管 ducts of lacrimal gland
10. 泪腺 lacrimal gland

图 8-47 右眶隔(前面观)
Right orbital septum
(anterior view)

1. 眶上神经和血管 supraorbital nerve and blood vessels
2. 滑车上神经 supratrochlear nerve
3. 上睑板 superior tarsus
4. 滑车下神经 infratrochlear nerve
5. 睑内侧韧带 medial palpebral ligament
6. 睑内侧连合 medial palpebral commissure
7. 下睑板 inferior tarsus
8. 眶隔 orbital septum
9. 睑外侧连合 lateral palpebral commissure
10. 睑外侧韧带 lateral palpebral ligament

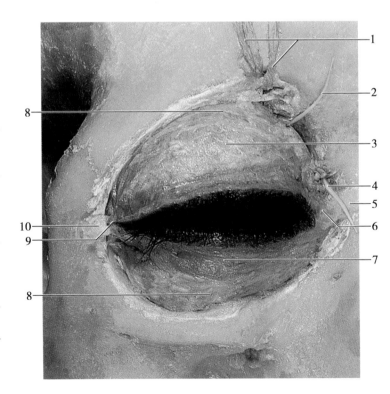

193

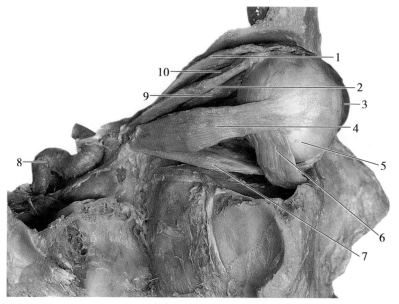

图 8-48　右眼球外肌(外侧面观)
Right extraocular muscles(lateral view)

1. 上睑提肌 levator palpebrae superioris
2. 上直肌 superior rectus
3. 角膜 cornea
4. 外直肌 lateral rectus
5. 眼球 eyeball
6. 下斜肌 inferior oblique
7. 下直肌 inferior rectus
8. 颈内动脉 internal carotid artery
9. 内直肌 medial rectus
10. 上斜肌 superior oblique

图 8-49　右眼球外肌(上面观)
Right extraocular muscles
(superior view)

1. 上睑提肌 levator palpebrae superioris
2. 上直肌 superior rectus
3. 外直肌 lateral rectus
4. 视神经(Ⅱ)optic nerve(Ⅱ)
5. 下直肌 inferior rectus
6. 内直肌 medial rectus
7. 上斜肌 superior oblique
8. 滑车 trochlea

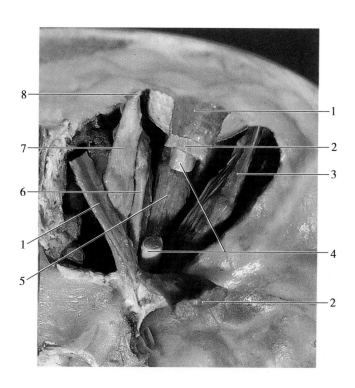

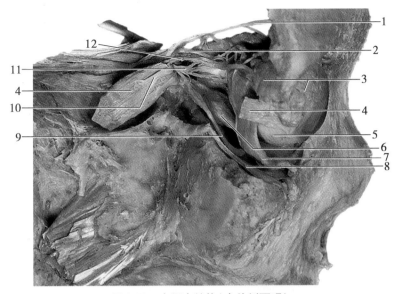

图 8-50 右眶内结构(右外侧面观)
Contents in right orbit(right lateral view)

1. 额神经 frontal nerve
2. 动眼神经(Ⅲ)上支 superior division of oculomotor nerve(Ⅲ)
3. 泪腺 lacrimal gland
4. 外直肌 lateral rectus
5. 眼球 eyeball
6. 下直肌 inferior rectus
7. 下斜肌 inferior oblique
8. 眶下神经 infraorbital nerve
9. 动眼神经(Ⅲ)下支 inferior division of oculomotor nerve(Ⅲ)
10. 展神经(Ⅵ)abducens nerve(Ⅵ)
11. 睫状神经节 ciliary ganglion
12. 泪腺神经 lacrimal nerve

图 8-51 右眼眶内容(上面观)
Contents in right orbital (superior view)

1. 额神经 frontal nerve
2. 泪腺 lacrimal gland
3. 上睑提肌 levator palpebrae superioris
4. 上直肌 superior rectus
5. 眼球 eyeball
6. 泪腺神经 lacrimal nerve
7. 外直肌 lateral rectus
8. 眼神经 ophthalmic nerve
9. 动眼神经(Ⅲ) oculomotor nerve(Ⅲ)
10. 展神经(Ⅵ) abducens nerve(Ⅵ)
11. 眼动脉 ophthalmic artery
12. 内直肌 medial rectus
13. 滑车上神经 supratrochlear nerve

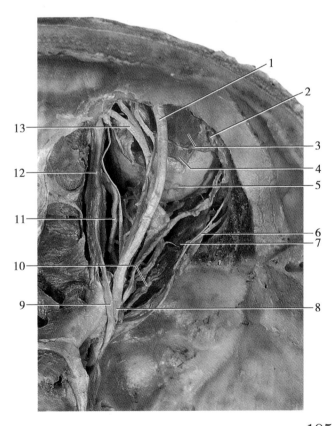

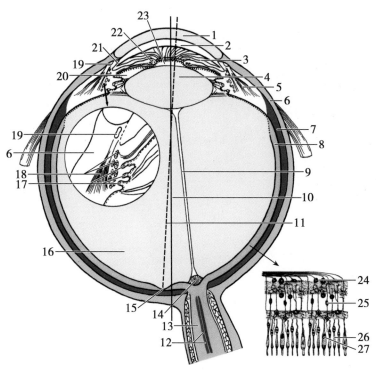

图 8-52　右眼球水平切面
模式图（下面观）
**Diagram for horizontal section
of left eyeball（inferior view）**

1. 角膜 cornea
2. 前房 anterior chamber
3. 虹膜 iris
4. 晶状体 lens
5. 睫状体 ciliary body
6. 巩膜 sclera
7. 脉络膜 choroid
8. 视网膜 retina
9. 玻璃体管 hyaloid canal
10. 眼轴 eye axis
11. 视轴 optic axis
12. 视网膜中央动脉和静脉
    central artery and vein of ret-
    ina
13. 视神经（Ⅱ）optic nerve（Ⅱ）
14. 视神经盘 optic disc
15. 黄斑 macula lutea
16. 玻璃体 vitreous body

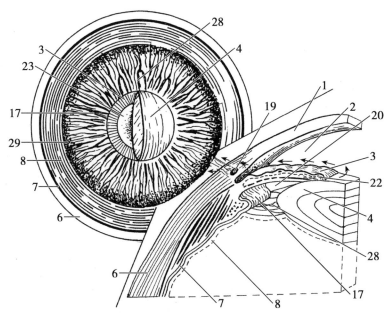

图 8-53　眼球前半模式图（后面观）
Diagram for anterior half of eyeball（posterior view）

17. 睫状突 ciliary processes
18. 睫状肌 ciliary muscle
19. 巩膜静脉窦 sinus venosus sclerae
20. 后房 posterior chamber
21. 前房角 anterior chamber angle
22. 瞳孔括约肌 sphincter pupillae
23. 瞳孔 pupil

24. 节细胞 ganglion cell
25. 双极细胞 bipolar cell
26. 视杆细胞 rod cell
27. 视锥细胞 cone cell
28. 睫状小带 ciliary zonule
29. 睫状环 ciliary ring

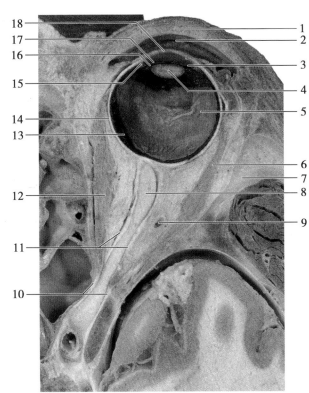

图 8-54 右眼眶水平断面(上面观)
Horizontal section through right orbit
(superior view)

1. 下睑 lower eyelid
2. 结膜囊 conjunctive sac
3. 虹膜 iris
4. 晶状体 lens
5. 视网膜 retina
6. 外直肌 lateral rectus
7. 眶脂体 adipose body of orbit
8. 视神经(Ⅱ) optic nerve(Ⅱ)
9. 眼动脉 ophthalmic artery
10. 总腱环 common tendinous ring
11. 视神经(Ⅱ)外鞘 outer sheath of optic nerve(Ⅱ)
12. 内直肌 medial rectus
13. 脉络膜 choroid
14. 巩膜 sclera
15. 睫状体 ciliary body
16. 后房 posterior chamber
17. 前房 anterior chamber
18. 角膜 cornea

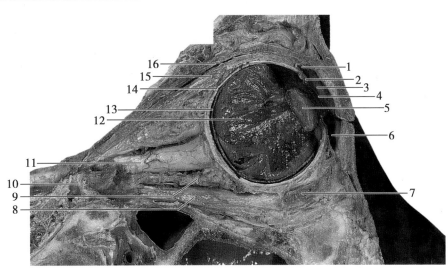

图 8-55 右眼球及眶矢状切面(外侧面观)
Sagittal section through right eyeball and orbital cavity(lateral view)

1. 结膜上穹 superior conjunctival fornix
2. 虹膜 iris
3. 睑结膜 palpebral conjunctiva
4. 角膜 cornea
5. 晶状体 lens
6. 结膜下穹 inferior conjunctival fornix
7. 下斜肌 inferior oblique
8. 下直肌 inferior rectus
9. 眶脂体 adipose body of orbit
10. 总腱环 common tendinous ring
11. 视神经(Ⅱ) optic nerve(Ⅱ)
12. 视网膜 retina
13. 脉络膜 choroid
14. 巩膜 sclera
15. 上直肌 superior rectus
16. 上睑提肌 levator palpebrae superioris

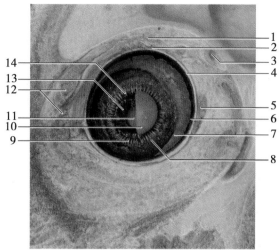

图 8-56　右眼球前半 (后面观)
**Anterior half of right eyeball
(posterior view)**

1. 上睑提肌 levator palpebrae superioris
2. 上直肌 superior rectus
3. 上斜肌腱 tendon of superior oblique
4. 巩膜 sclera
5. 内直肌 medial rectus
6. 脉络膜 choroid
7. 视网膜 retina
8. 睫状缘 ciliary margin
9. 睫状襞 ciliary folds
10. 晶状体 lens
11. 瞳孔 pupil
12. 泪腺 lacrimal gland
13. 虹膜 iris
14. 睫状突 ciliary process

图 8-57　眼底血管 (活体眼底镜照片)
Fundus photograph of right eye

1. 视网膜颞侧上小静脉 superior temporal venule of retina
2. 视网膜颞侧上小动脉 superior temporal arteriole of retina
3. 视网膜鼻侧上小动脉 superior nasal arteriole of retina
4. 视网膜鼻侧上小静脉 superior nasal venule of retina
5. 视神经盘 optic disc
6. 视网膜鼻侧下小静脉 inferior nasal venule of retina
7. 视网膜鼻侧下小动脉 inferior nasal arteriole of retina
8. 视网膜颞侧下小动脉 inferior temporal arteriole of retina
9. 视网膜颞侧下小静脉 inferior temporal venule of retina
10. 黄斑下小静脉 inferior macular venule
11. 黄斑下小动脉 inferior macular arteriole
12. 黄斑 macula lutea
13. 黄斑上小静脉 superior macular venule
14. 黄斑上小动脉 superior macula arteriole

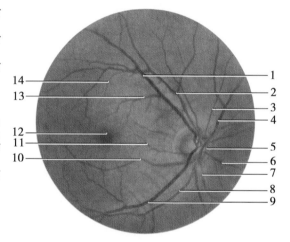

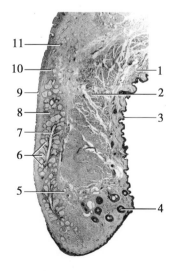

图 8-58　上眼睑切片 Section of upper eyelid

1. 皮下组织 subcutaneous tissue
2. 眼轮匝肌 orbicularis oculi
3. 皮肤 skin
4. 毛囊 hair follicle
5. 下动脉弓 inferior arterial arch
6. 睑板腺 tarsal glands
7. 睑板腺管 tarsal gland ducts
8. 睑板 tarsus
9. 睑结膜 palpebral conjunctiva
10. 米勒肌 Müller muscle
11. 上动脉弓 superior arterial arch

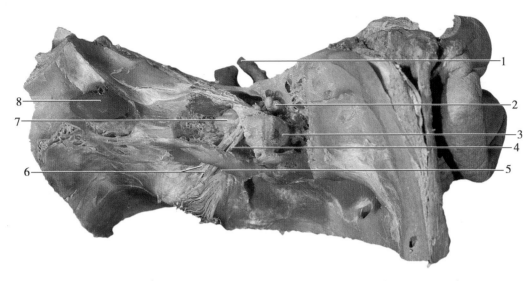

图 8-59　右前庭蜗器（上面观）**Right vestibulocochlear organ（superior view）**

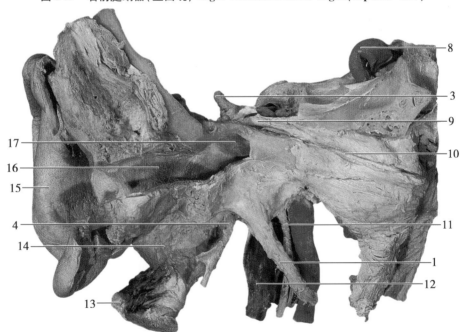

图 8-60　右前庭蜗器（前面观）**Right vestibulocochlear organ（anterior view）**

1. 颞骨茎突 styloid process of temporal bone
2. 听小骨 auditory ossicles
3. 骨半规管 bony semicircular canals
4. 面神经（Ⅶ）facial nerve（Ⅶ）
5. 内耳门 internal acoustic pore
6. 前庭蜗神经（Ⅷ）vestibulocochlear nerve（Ⅷ）
7. 耳蜗 cochlea
8. 颈内动脉 internal carotid artery
9. 鼓膜张肌 tensor tympani
10. 咽鼓管 pharyngotympanic tube
11. 迷走神经（Ⅹ）vagus nerve（Ⅹ）
12. 颈内静脉 internal jugular vein
13. 胸锁乳突肌 sternocleidomastoid
14. 颞骨乳突 mastoid process of temporal bone
15. 耳廓 auricle
16. 外耳道 external acoustic meatus
17. 鼓膜 tympanic membrane

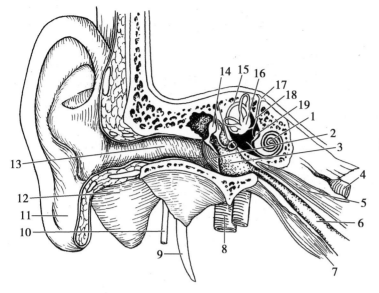

图 8-61 右前庭蜗器模
式图（前面观）
**Diagram of right vestibulocochlear
organ（anterior view）**

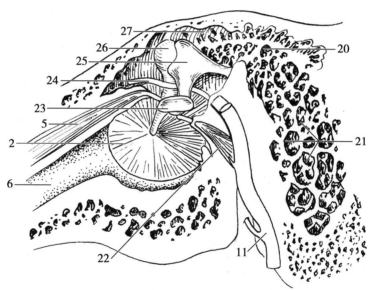

图 8-62 右鼓室外侧壁模式图（内侧面观）
Diagram for lateral wall of right tympanic cavity（medial view）

1. 耳蜗 cochlea
2. 鼓膜 tympanic membrane
3. 鼓室 tympanic cavity
4. 颈内动脉 internal carotid artery
5. 鼓膜张肌 tensor tympani
6. 咽鼓管 pharyngotympanic tube
7. 腭帆提肌 levator veli palatini
8. 颈内静脉 internal jugular vein
9. 颞骨茎突 styloid process of temporal bone
10. 面神经（Ⅶ）facial nerve（Ⅶ）
11. 耳垂 auricular lobule
12. 颞骨乳突 mastoid process of temporal bone
13. 外耳道 external acoustic meatus
14. 听小骨 auditory ossicles
15. 骨半规管 bony semicircular canals
16. 椭圆囊 utricle
17. 内淋巴囊 endolymphatic sac
18. 内淋巴管 endolymphatic duct
19. 球囊 saccule
20. 乳突窦 mastoid antrum
21. 乳突小房 mastoid cells
22. 镫骨肌 stapedius
23. 镫骨 stapes
24. 鼓索 chorda tympanic
25. 砧骨 incus
26. 锤骨 malleus
27. 鼓室上隐窝 epitympanic recess

200

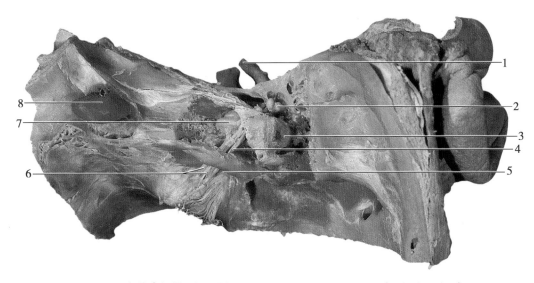

图 8-59 右前庭蜗器（上面观）**Right vestibulocochlear organ（superior view）**

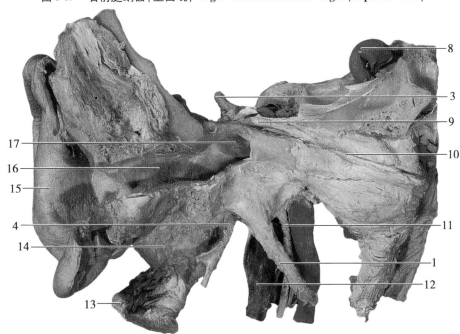

图 8-60 右前庭蜗器（前面观）**Right vestibulocochlear organ（anterior view）**

1. 颞骨茎突 styloid process of temporal bone
2. 听小骨 auditory ossicles
3. 骨半规管 bony semicircular canals
4. 面神经（Ⅶ） facial nerve（Ⅶ）
5. 内耳门 internal acoustic pore
6. 前庭蜗神经（Ⅷ） vestibulocochlear nerve（Ⅷ）
7. 耳蜗 cochlea
8. 颈内动脉 internal carotid artery
9. 鼓膜张肌 tensor tympani
10. 咽鼓管 pharyngotympanic tube
11. 迷走神经（Ⅹ） vagus nerve（Ⅹ）
12. 颈内静脉 internal jugular vein
13. 胸锁乳突肌 sternocleidomastoid
14. 颞骨乳突 mastoid process of temporal bone
15. 耳廓 auricle
16. 外耳道 external acoustic meatus
17. 鼓膜 tympanic membrane

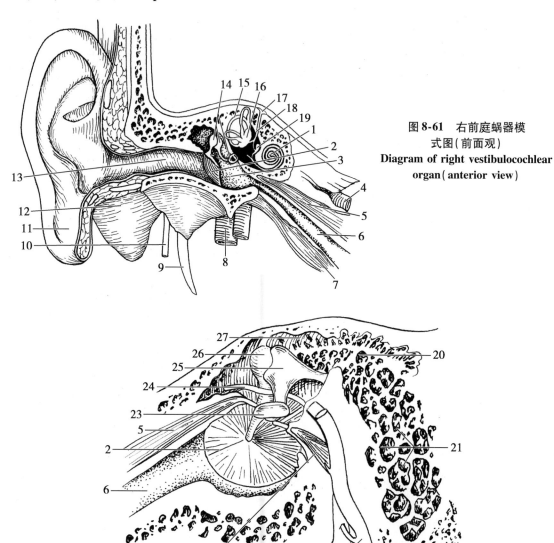

图 8-61 右前庭蜗器模
式图(前面观)
**Diagram of right vestibulocochlear
organ(anterior view)**

图 8-62 右鼓室外侧壁模式图(内侧面观)
Diagram for lateral wall of right tympanic cavity(medial view)

1. 耳蜗 cochlea
2. 鼓膜 tympanic membrane
3. 鼓室 tympanic cavity
4. 颈内动脉 internal carotid artery
5. 鼓膜张肌 tensor tympani
6. 咽鼓管 pharyngotympanic tube
7. 腭帆提肌 levator veli palatini
8. 颈内静脉 internal jugular vein
9. 颞骨茎突 styloid process of temporal bone
10. 面神经(Ⅶ) facial nerve(Ⅶ)
11. 耳垂 auricular lobule
12. 颞骨乳突 mastoid process of temporal bone
13. 外耳道 external acoustic meatus
14. 听小骨 auditory ossicles
15. 骨半规管 bony semicircular canals
16. 椭圆囊 utricle
17. 内淋巴囊 endolymphatic sac
18. 内淋巴管 endolymphatic duct
19. 球囊 saccule
20. 乳突窦 mastoid antrum
21. 乳突小房 mastoid cells
22. 镫骨肌 stapedius
23. 镫骨 stapes
24. 鼓索 chorda tympanic
25. 砧骨 incus
26. 锤骨 malleus
27. 鼓室上隐窝 epitympanic recess

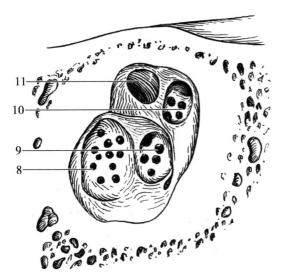

图 8-63　右内耳道底模式图（内侧面观）
Diagram for bottom of right internal acoustic meatus（medial view）

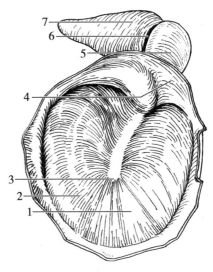

图 8-64　右鼓膜模式图（外侧观）
Diagram for right tympanic membrane （lateral view）

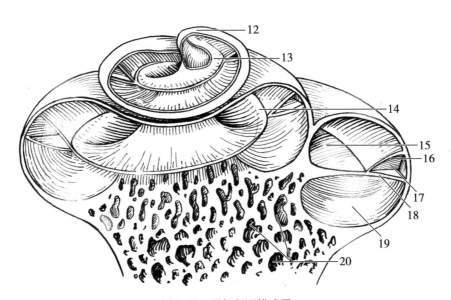

图 8-65　耳蜗断面模式图
Diagram for section through cochlea

1. 光锥 cone of light
2. 鼓膜紧张部 pars tensa of tympanic membrane
3. 鼓膜脐 umbo of tympanic membrane
4. 鼓膜松弛部 pars flaccida of tympanic membrane
5. 锤骨头 head of malleus
6. 砧锤关节 incudomalleolar joint
7. 砧骨体 body of incus
8. 蜗区 cochlear area
9. 前庭下区 inferior vestibular area
10. 前庭上区 superior vestibular area

11. 面神经区 area of facial nerve
12. 蜗顶 cupula of cochlea
13. 螺旋板钩 hamulus of spiral lamina
14. 骨螺旋板 osseous spiral lamina
15. 前庭阶 scala vestibule
16. 前庭膜 vestibular membrane
17. 蜗管 cochlear duct
18. 螺旋膜 spiral membrane
19. 鼓阶 scala tympani
20. 蜗轴 cochlear axis

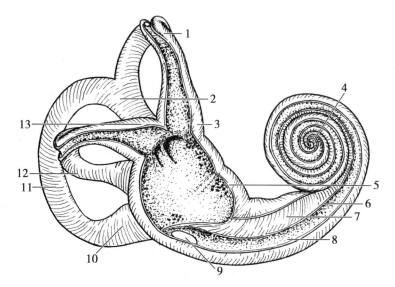

图 8-66 右骨迷路内面模式图
Diagram for interior of right bony labyrinth

1. 前骨半规管 anterior bony semicircular canal
2. 总骨脚 bony crus commune
3. 前骨壶腹 anterior bony ampulla
4. 蜗顶 cupula of cochlea
5. 前庭 vestibule
6. 骨螺旋板 osseous spiral lamina
7. 前庭阶 scala vestibule

8. 鼓阶 scala tympani
9. 蜗窗（圆窗）fenestra cochleae（round window）
10. 后骨壶腹 posterior bony ampulla
11. 后骨半规管 posterior bony semicircular canal
12. 外骨半规管 lateral bony semicircular canal
13. 外骨壶腹 lateral bony ampulla

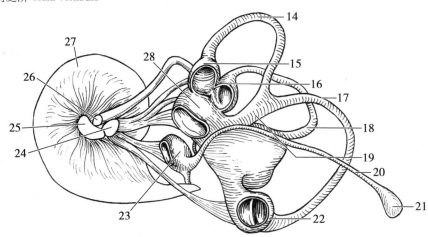

图 8-67 右膜迷路模式图 Diagram for right membranous labyrinty

14. 前膜半规管 anterior membranous semicircular duct
15. 前膜壶腹 anterior membranous ampulla
16. 外膜壶腹 lateral membranous ampulla
17. 后膜半规管 posterior membranous semicircular duct
18. 外膜半规管 lateral membranous semicircular duct
19. 总膜脚 membranous crus commune
20. 内淋巴管 endolymphatic duct
21. 内淋巴囊 endolymphatic sac

22. 后膜壶腹 posterior membranous ampulla
23. 球囊 saccule
24. 前庭神经 vestibular nerve
25. 蜗神经 cochlear nerve
26. 面神经（Ⅶ）facial nerve（Ⅶ）
27. 蜗管 cochlear duct
28. 椭圆囊 utricle

202

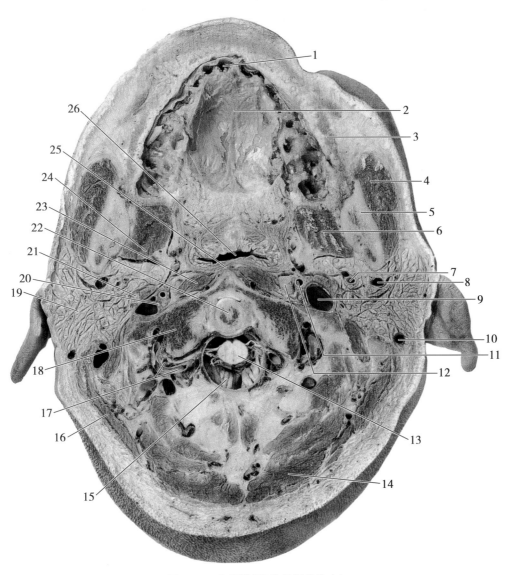

图 8-68 头部横断面(经枢椎齿突)
Transverse section through head at level of dens of axis

1. 上颌骨牙槽突 superior alveolar process of maxilla
2. 硬腭 hard palate
3. 颊肌 buccinator
4. 咬肌 masseter
5. 下颌支 ramus of mandible
6. 翼内肌 medial pterygoid
7. 颈外动脉 external carotid artery
8. 下颌后静脉 retromandibular vein
9. 颈内静脉 internal jugular vein
10. 耳后静脉 posterior auricular vein
11. 颈内动脉 internal carotid artery
12. 交感干颈上神经节 superior cervical ganglion of sympathetic trunk
13. 脊髓 spinal cord
14. 斜方肌 trapezius
15. 小脑 cerebellum
16. 胸锁乳突肌 sternocleidomastoid
17. 椎动脉和静脉 vertebral artery and vein
18. 寰椎 atlas
19. 腮腺 parotid gland
20. 迷走神经(Ⅹ) vagus nerve(Ⅹ)
21. 颞骨茎突 styloid process of temporal bone
22. 枢椎齿突 dens of axis
23. 头长肌 longus capitis
24. 翼外肌 lateral pterygoid
25. 咽上缩肌 superior pharyngeal constrictor
26. 咽 pharynx

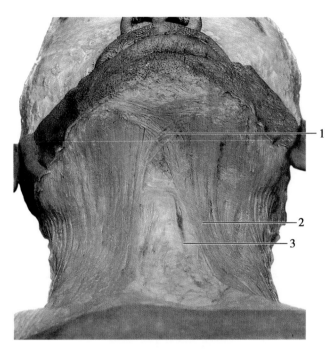

图 8-69 颈阔肌(前面观)
Platysma(anterior view)

1. 颈阔肌交叉纤维 cross fibers of platysma
2. 颈阔肌 platysma
3. 颈前静脉 anterior jugular vein

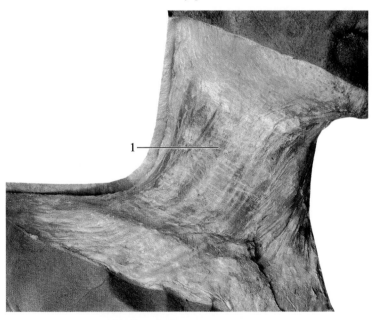

图 8-70 颈阔肌(右前外侧面观)
Platysma(right anterolateral view)
1. 颈阔肌 platysma

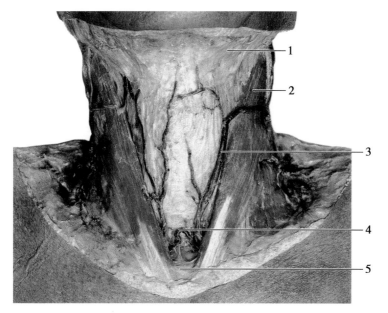

图 8-71　颈浅静脉（Ⅰ）（前面观）
Superficial veins of neck（Ⅰ）（anterior view）

1. 颈深筋膜浅层 superficial layer of cervical deep fascia
2. 胸锁乳突肌 sternocleidomastoid
3. 颈前静脉 anterior jugular vein
4. 颈静脉弓 jugular venous arch
5. 胸骨上窝 suprasternal fossa

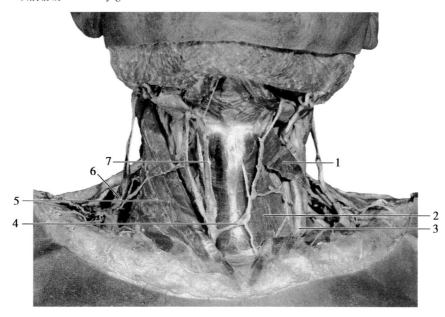

图 8-72　颈浅静脉（Ⅱ）（前面观）
Superficial veins of neck（Ⅱ）（anterior view）

1. 肩胛舌骨肌 omohyoid
2. 胸骨舌骨肌 sternohyoid
3. 颈内静脉 internal jugular vein
4. 颈静脉弓 jugular venous arch
5. 胸锁乳突肌 sternocleidomastoid
6. 颈外静脉 external jugular vein
7. 颈前静脉 anterior jugular vein

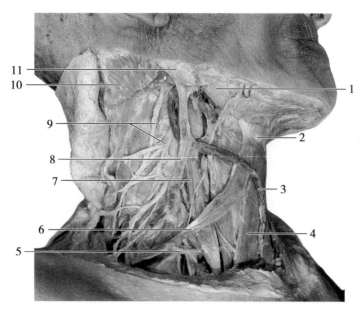

图 8-73 颈丛和颈浅静脉(右外侧面观)
Cervical plexus and superficial jugular veins(right lateral view)

1. 下颌下腺 submandibular gland
2. 舌骨 hyoid bone
3. 颈前静脉 anterior jugular vein
4. 胸骨舌骨肌 sternohyoid
5. 颈横动脉 transverse cervical artery
6. 肩胛舌骨肌 omohyoid
7. 颈内静脉 internal jugular vein
8. 颈外静脉 external jugular vein
9. 颈丛 cervical plexus
10. 胸锁乳突肌 sternocleidomastoid
11. 腮腺 parotid gland

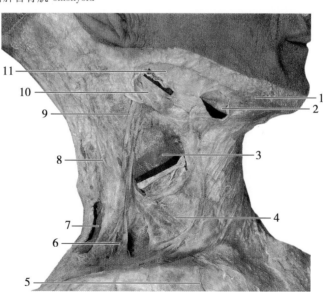

图 8-74 颈深筋膜浅层(右外侧面观)
Superficial layer of cervical deep fascia(right lateral view)

1. 颈阔肌 platysma
2. 下颌下腺 submandibular gland
3. 胸锁乳突肌 sternocleidomastoid
4. 颈深筋膜浅层 superficial layer of cervical deep fascia
5. 锁骨上神经 supraclavicular nerve
6. 颈外静脉 external jugular vein
7. 斜方肌 trapezius
8. 枕小神经 lesser occipital nerve
9. 耳大神经 great auricular nerve
10. 腮腺 parotid gland
11. 腮腺筋膜 parotid fascia

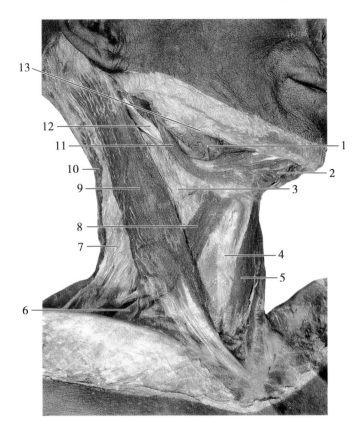

图 8-75 颈部三角（右前外侧面观）
Triangles of neck（right anterolateral view）

1. 下颌下三角 submandibular triangle
2. 颏下三角 submental triangle
3. 颈动脉三角 carotid triangle
4. 肌三角 muscular triangle
5. 胸骨舌骨肌 sternohyoid
6. 锁骨上大窝 greater supraclavicular fossa
7. 枕三角 occipital triangle
8. 肩胛舌骨肌上腹 superior belly of omohyoid
9. 胸锁乳突肌 sternocleidomastoid
10. 斜方肌 trapezius
11. 茎突舌骨肌 stylohyoid
12. 二腹肌后腹 posterior belly of digastric
13. 下颌骨下缘 inferior margin of mandible

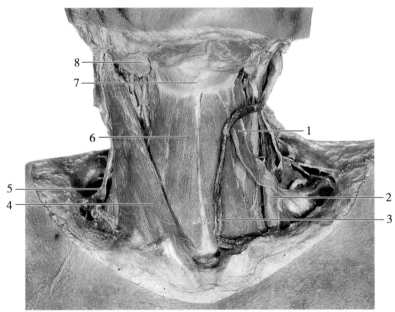

图 8-76 颈前区肌（前面观）
Muscles of anterior cervical region（anterior view）

1. 肩胛舌骨肌 omohyoid
2. 颈内静脉 internal jugular vein
3. 颈前静脉 anterior jugular vein
4. 胸锁乳突肌 sternocleidomastoid
5. 颈外静脉 external jugular vein
6. 胸骨舌骨肌 sternohyoid
7. 舌骨 hyoid bone
8. 下颌下腺 submandibular gland

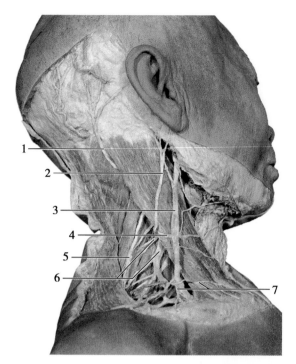

图 8-77　颈丛分支（右外侧面观）
Branches of cervical plexus
（right lateral view）

1. 枕小神经 lesser occipital nerve
2. 耳大神经 great auricular nerve
3. 颈外静脉 external jugular vein
4. 颈横神经 transverse cervical nerve
5. 副神经（Ⅺ）accessory nerve（Ⅺ）
6. 颈丛 cervical plexus
7. 锁骨上神经 supraclavicular nerve

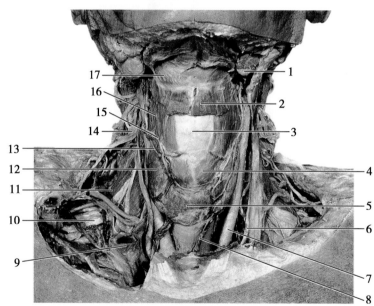

图 8-78　甲状腺区（前面观）Region of thyroid gland（anterior view）

1. 下颌下腺 submandibular gland
2. 胸骨舌骨肌 sternohyoid
3. 甲状软骨 thyroid cartilage
4. 环甲肌 cricothyroid
5. 甲状腺峡部 isthmus of thyroid gland
6. 迷走神经（Ⅹ）vagus nerve（Ⅹ）
7. 颈总动脉 common carotid artery
8. 甲状腺下静脉 inferior thyroid vein
9. 颈内静脉 internal jugular vein
10. 臂丛 brachial plexus
11. 中斜角肌 scalenus medius
12. 甲状腺侧叶 lateral lobe of thyroid gland
13. 喉上神经 superior laryngeal nerve
14. 颈丛 cervical plexus
15. 甲状腺上动脉 superior thyroid artery
16. 甲状舌骨肌 thyrohyoid
17. 下颌舌骨肌 mylohyoid

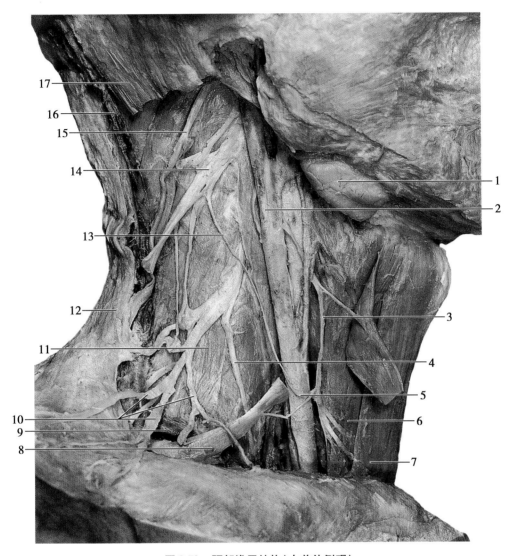

图 8-79 颈部浅层结构(右前外侧观)
Superficial layer of structures of neck(right anterolateral view)

1. 下颌下腺 submandibular gland
2. 颈内静脉 internal jugular vein
3. 颈襻上根 superior root of ansa cervicalis
4. 膈神经 phrenic nerve
5. 颈襻 ansa cervicalis
6. 胸骨甲状肌 sternothyroid
7. 胸骨舌骨肌 sternohyoid
8. 肩胛舌骨肌 omohyoid
9. 锁骨下静脉 subclavian vein
10. 锁骨上神经 supraclavicular nerve
11. 肩胛提肌 levator scapulae
12. 斜方肌 trapezius
13. 颈襻下根 inferior root of ansa cervicalis
14. 颈丛 cervical plexus
15. 副神经(XI) accessory nerve(XI)
16. 枕静脉 occipital vein
17. 胸锁乳突肌 sternocleidomastoid

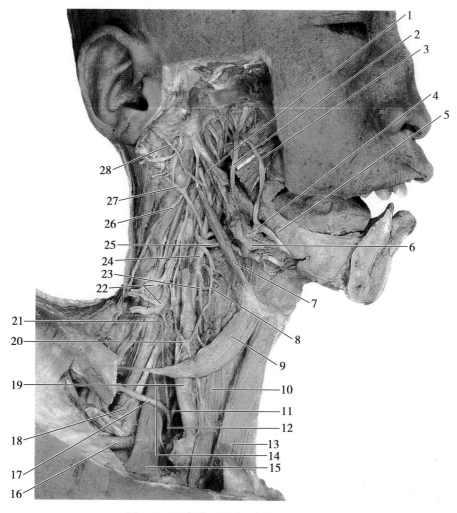

图 8-80 颈部中层结构(右前外侧面观)
Middle layer of structures of neck(right anterolateral view)

1. 舌咽神经(Ⅸ) glossopharyngeal nerve(Ⅸ)
2. 下牙槽神经 inferior alveolar nerve
3. 舌神经 lingual nerve
4. 下颌下节 submandibular ganglion
5. 舌下腺 sublingual gland
6. 下颌下腺 submandibular gland
7. 茎突舌骨肌 stylohyoid
8. 颈襻上根 superior root of ansa cervicalis
9. 肩胛舌骨肌 omohyoid
10. 胸骨甲状肌 sternothyroid
11. 甲状腺下动脉 inferior thyroid artery
12. 甲状颈干 thyrocervical trunk
13. 胸骨舌骨肌 sternohyoid
14. 膈神经 phrenic nerve
15. 前斜角肌 scalenus anterior
16. 锁骨下动脉 subclavian artery
17. 颈横动脉 transverse cervical artery
18. 臂丛 brachial plexus
19. 颈内静脉 internal jugular vein
20. 颈襻 ansa cervicalis
21. 颈襻下根 inferior root of ansa cervicalis
22. 颈丛 cervical plexus
23. 甲状腺上动脉 superior thyroid artery
24. 颈外动脉 external carotid artery
25. 舌下神经(Ⅻ) hypoglossal nerve(Ⅻ)
26. 副神经(Ⅺ) accessory nerve(Ⅺ)
27. 枕动脉 occipital artery
28. 耳后动脉 posterior auricular artery

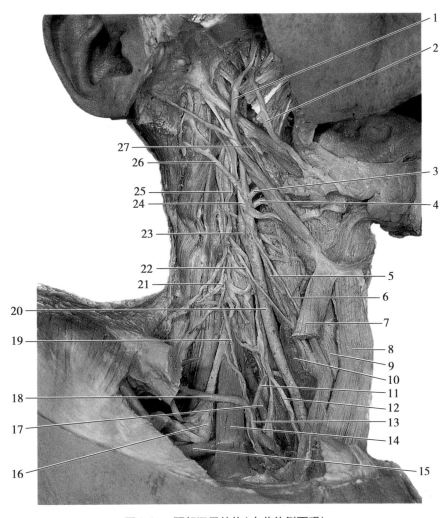

图 8-81 颈部深层结构(右前外侧面观)
Deep layer of structures of neck(right anterolateral view)

1. 下牙槽神经 inferior alveolar nerve
2. 舌神经 lingual nerve
3. 面动脉 facial artery
4. 舌动脉 lingual artery
5. 甲状腺上动脉 superior thyroid artery
6. 颈襻上根 superior root of ansa cervicalis
7. 肩胛舌骨肌 omohyoid
8. 胸骨舌骨肌 sternohyoid
9. 胸骨甲状肌 sternothyroid
10. 甲状腺 thyroid gland
11. 甲状腺下动脉 inferior thyroid artery
12. 迷走神经(Ⅹ) vagus nerve(Ⅹ)
13. 甲状颈干 thyrocervical trunk
14. 前斜角肌 scalenus anterior
15. 锁骨下动脉 subclavian artery
16. 臂丛 brachial plexus
17. 椎动脉 vertebral artery
18. 颈横动脉 transverse cervical artery
19. 膈神经 phrenic nerve
20. 颈总动脉 common carotid artery
21. 颈丛 cervical plexus
22. 颈襻下根 inferior root of ansa cervicalis
23. 颈动脉窦 carotid sinus
24. 舌下神经(Ⅻ) hypoglossal nerve(Ⅻ)
25. 副神经(Ⅺ) accessory nerve(Ⅺ)
26. 枕动脉 occipital artery
27. 舌咽神经(Ⅸ) glossopharyngeal nerve(Ⅸ)

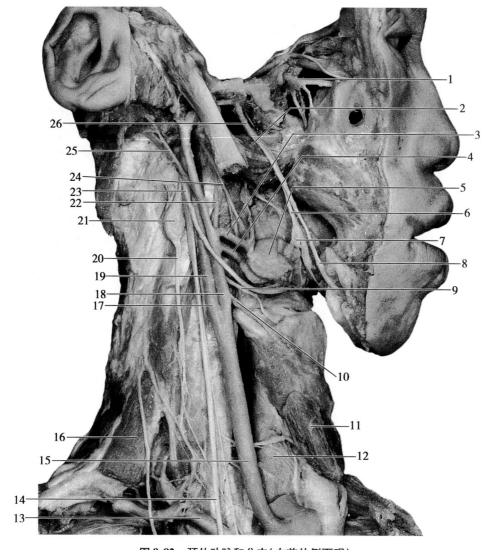

图 8-82　颈外动脉和分支 (右前外侧面观)
External carotid artery and its branches (right anterolateral view)

1. 上颌神经 maxillary nerve
2. 翼外肌 lateral pterygoid
3. 面动脉 facial artery
4. 舌动脉 lingual artery
5. 下颌下腺 submandibular gland
6. 舌神经 lingual nerve
7. 下颌下节 submandibular ganglion
8. 下牙槽神经 inferior alveolar nerve
9. 喉上神经 superior laryngeal nerve
10. 甲状腺上动脉 superior thyroid artery
11. 甲状腺 thyroid gland
12. 咽 pharynx
13. 锁骨下动脉 subclavian artery
14. 迷走神经 (X) vagus nerve (X)

15. 颈总动脉 common carotid artery
16. 斜方肌 trapezius
17. 颈动脉窦 carotid sinus
18. 颈外动脉 external carotid artery
19. 颈内动脉 internal carotid artery
20. 交感干 sympathetic trunk
21. 交感干颈上神经节 superior cervical ganglion of sympathetic trunk
22. 咽升动脉 ascending pharyngeal artery
23. 舌下神经 (XII) hypoglossal nerve (XII)
24. 舌咽神经 (IX) glossopharyngeal nerve (IX)
25. 枕动脉 occipital artery
26. 下颌神经 mandibular nerve

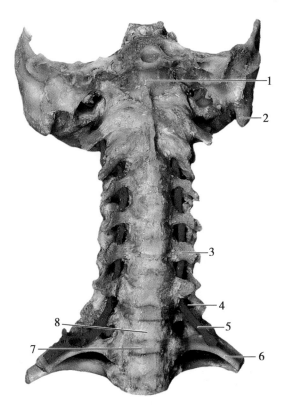

图 8-83 椎动脉和颈椎(前面观)
**Vertebral artery and cervical vertebrae
(anterior view)**

1. 枕骨 occipital bone
2. 颞骨乳突 mastoid process of temporal bone
3. 颈椎横突 transverse process of a cervical vertebra
4. 颈椎横突孔 transverse foramen of a cervical vertebra
5. 椎动脉 vertebral artery
6. 第一肋 first rib
7. 颈椎椎体 body of a cervical vertebra
8. 椎间盘 intervertebral disc

图 8-84 椎动脉和颈椎(左外侧面观)
**Vertebral artery and cervical vertebrae
(left lateral view)**

1. 外耳道 external acoustic meatus
2. 颞骨乳突 mastoid process of temporal bone
3. 枕骨 occipital bone
4. 项韧带 ligamentum nuchae
5. 椎动脉 vertebral artery
6. 第七颈椎棘突 spinous process of seventh cervical
vertebra

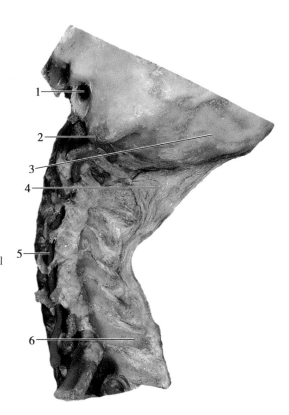

213

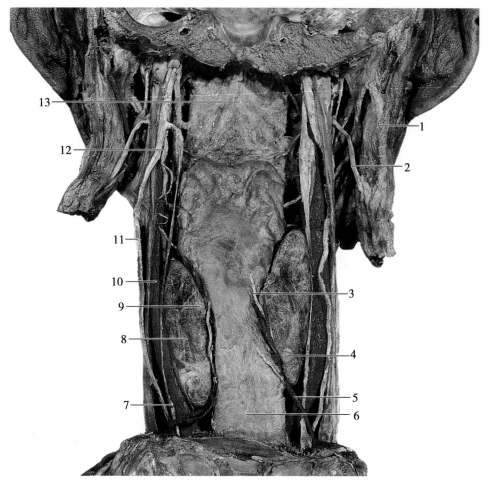

图 8-85　甲状腺区(后面观)
Region of thyroid gland(posterior view)

1. 胸锁乳突肌 sternocleidomastoid
2. 副神经(XI) accessory nerve(XI)
3. 右喉返神经 right recurrent laryngeal nerve
4. 下甲状旁腺 interior parathyroid gland
5. 甲状腺下动脉 inferior thyroid artery
6. 食管颈部 cervical part of esophagus
7. 迷走神经(X)颈心支 cervical cardiac branch of vagus nerve(X)
8. 甲状腺 thyroid gland
9. 上甲状旁腺 superior parathyroid gland
10. 颈总动脉 common carotid artery
11. 迷走神经(X) vagus nerve(X)
12. 喉上神经 superior laryngeal nerve
13. 咽 pharynx

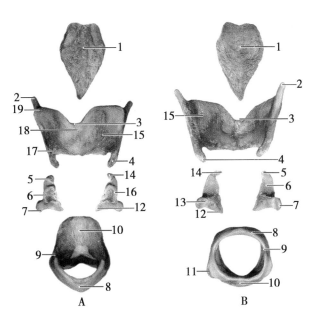

图 8-86　喉软骨
Cartilages of larynx

A. 前面观 Anterior view
B. 后面观 Posterior view

1. 会厌软骨 epiglottis
2. 甲状软骨上角 superior cornu of thyroid cartilage
3. 甲状切迹 thyroid notch
4. 甲状软骨下角 inferior cornu of thyroid cartilage
5. 杓状软骨尖 apex of arytenoid cartilage
6. 杓状软骨 arytenoid cartilage
7. 杓状软骨肌突 muscular process of arytenoid cartilage
8. 环状软骨弓 arch of cricoid cartilage
9. 环状软骨 cricoid cartilage
10. 环状软骨板 lamina of cricoid cartilage
11. 甲关节面 thyroid articular surface
12. 杓状软骨声带突 vocal process of arytenoid cartilage
13. 杓状软骨关节面 articular surface of arytenoid cartilage
14. 小角软骨 corniculate cartilage
15. 甲状软骨板 lamina of thyroid cartilage
16. 弓状嵴 arcuate crest
17. 下结节 inferior thyroid tubercle
18. 喉结 laryngeal prominence
19. 上结节 superior thyroid tubercle

图 8-87　喉软骨和韧带
Cartilages and ligaments of larynx

A. 前面观 Anterior view
B. 后面观 Posterior view

1. 会厌软骨 epiglottis
2. 舌骨大角 greater cornu of hyoid bone
3. 甲状舌骨膜 thyrohyoid membrane
4. 甲状软骨 thyroid cartilage
5. 杓状软骨 arytenoid cartilage
6. 杓状软骨肌突 muscular process of arytenoid cartilage
7. 环状软骨板 lamina of cricoid cartilage
8. 气管软骨 tracheal cartilages
9. 甲状软骨下角 inferior cornu of thyroid cartilage
10. 杓状软骨声带突 vocal process of arytenoid cartilage
11. 小角软骨 corniculate cartilage
12. 甲状软骨上角 superior cornu of thyroid cartilage
13. 舌骨体 body of hyoid bone
14. 甲状舌骨正中韧带 median thyrohyoid ligament
15. 甲状切迹 thyroid notch
16. 喉结 laryngeal prominence
17. 环状软骨 cricoid cartilage
18. 环韧带 annular ligament
19. 环甲韧带 cricothyroid ligament

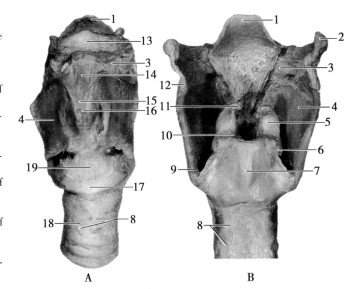

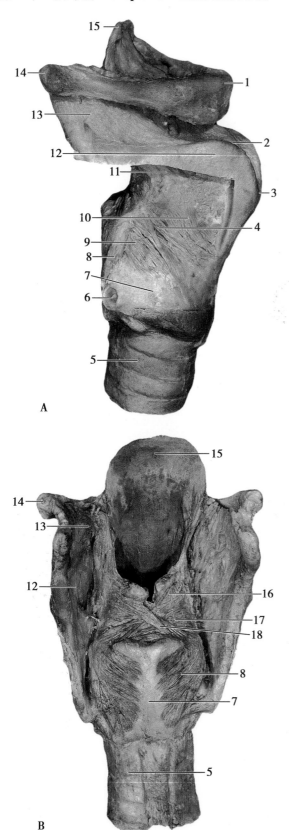

A

B

图 8-88 喉肌 Muscles of larynx

A. 右外侧面观 Right lateral view

B. 后面观 Posterior view

1. 舌骨体 body of hyoid bone
2. 甲状切迹 thyroid notch
3. 喉结 laryngeal prominence
4. 甲杓肌 thyroarytenoid
5. 气管软骨 tracheal cartilage
6. 甲关节面 thyroid articular surface
7. 环状软骨 cricoid cartilage
8. 环杓后肌 posterior cricoarytenoid
9. 环杓侧肌 lateral cricoarytenoid
10. 甲会厌肌 thyroepiglotticus
11. 方形膜 quadrangular membrane
12. 甲状软骨板 lamina of thyroid cartilage
13. 甲状舌骨膜 thyrohyoid membrane
14. 舌骨大角 greater cornu of hyoid bone
15. 会厌 epiglottis
16. 杓会厌肌 aryepiglotticus
17. 杓横肌 transverse arytenoid
18. 杓斜肌 oblique arytenoid

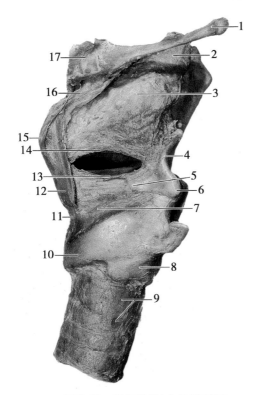

图 8-89　喉纤维膜（右外侧面观）
Fibrous membranes of larynx (right lateral view)

1. 舌骨大角 greater cornu of hyoid bone
2. 会厌 epiglottis
3. 方形膜 quadrangular membrane
4. 杓状软骨尖 apex of arytenoid cartilage
5. 杓状软骨声带突 vocal process of arytenoid cartilage
6. 杓状软骨肌突 muscular process of arytenoid cartilage
7. 弹性圆锥 conus elasticus
8. 环状软骨板 lamina of cricoid cartilage
9. 气管软骨 tracheal cartilage
10. 环状软骨弓 arch of cricoid cartilage
11. 环甲韧带 cricothyroid ligament
12. 甲状软骨 thyroid cartilage
13. 声韧带 vocal ligament
14. 前庭韧带 vestibular ligament
15. 喉结 laryngeal prominence
16. 甲舌膜 thyrohyoid membrane
17. 舌骨体 body of hyoid bone
18. 杓会厌襞 aryepiglottic fold
19. 梨状隐窝 piriform recess
20. 前庭襞 vestibular fold
21. 声襞 vocal fold
22. 声门下腔 infraglottic cavity
23. 喉前庭 laryngeal vestibule

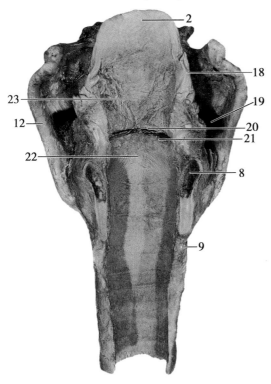

图 8-90　喉腔（后面观）
Cavity of larynx (posterior view)

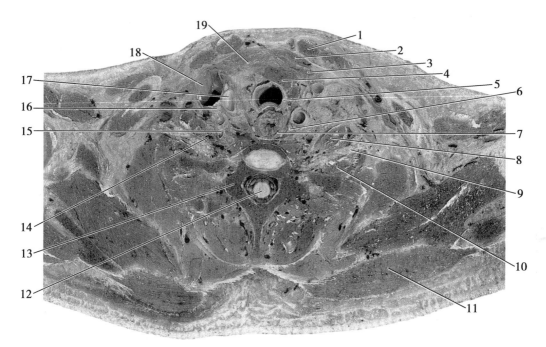

图 8-91 经第七颈椎间盘颈部横断面（下面观）
Transverse section through neck at level of seventh cervical vertebral disc (inferior view)

1. 胸锁乳突肌 sternocleidomastoid
2. 胸骨舌骨肌 sternohyoid
3. 肩胛舌骨肌 omohyoid
4. 甲状腺 thyroid gland
5. 气管 trachea
6. 左喉返神经 left recurrent laryngeal nerve
7. 食管 esophagus
8. 前斜角肌 scalenus anterior
9. 臂丛 brachial plexus
10. 中斜角肌 scalenus medius
11. 斜方肌 trapezius
12. 脊髓 spinal cord
13. 第七颈椎 seventh cervical vertebra
14. 椎静脉 vertebral vein
15. 椎动脉 vertebral artery
16. 迷走神经（Ⅹ）vagus nerve（Ⅹ）
17. 颈总动脉 common carotid artery
18. 颈内静脉 internal jugular vein
19. 胸骨甲状肌 sternothyroid

第 9 章　中枢神经系统

Chapter 9　Central Nervous System

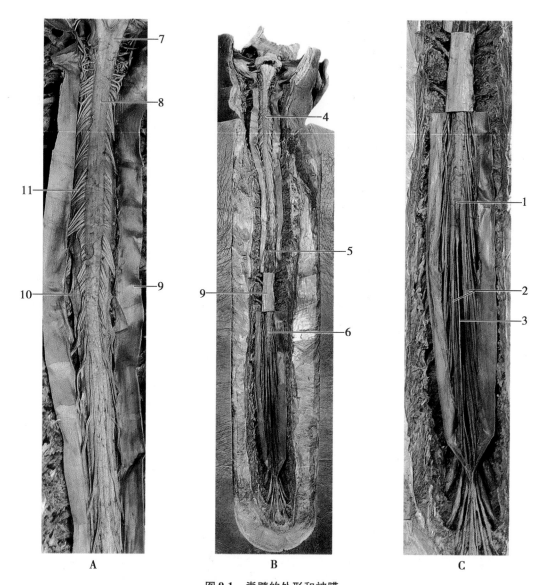

A　　　　　　　　　　B　　　　　　　　　　C

图 9-1　脊髓的外形和被膜
External features and meninges of the spinal cord

A. 颈胸段, 后面观 Cervicothoracic part, posterior view
B. 全长, 后面观 Whole length, posterior view
C. 腰骶段, 后面观 Lumbosacral part, posterior view

1. 脊髓圆锥 conus medullaris
2. 马尾 cauda equina
3. 终丝 filum terminale
4. 颈膨大 cervical enlargement
5. 脊髓蛛网膜 spinal arachnoid mater
6. 腰骶膨大 lumbosacral enlargement

7. 延髓 medulla oblongata
8. 背正中沟 dorsal median sulcus
9. 硬脊膜 spinal dura mater
10. 齿状韧带 denticulate ligament
11. 后根 posterior root

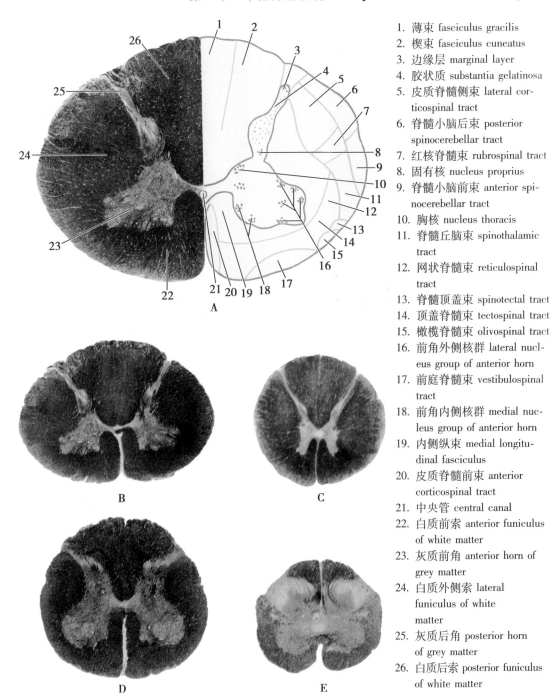

1. 薄束 fasciculus gracilis
2. 楔束 fasciculus cuneatus
3. 边缘层 marginal layer
4. 胶状质 substantia gelatinosa
5. 皮质脊髓侧束 lateral corticospinal tract
6. 脊髓小脑后束 posterior spinocerebellar tract
7. 红核脊髓束 rubrospinal tract
8. 固有核 nucleus proprius
9. 脊髓小脑前束 anterior spinocerebellar tract
10. 胸核 nucleus thoracis
11. 脊髓丘脑束 spinothalamic tract
12. 网状脊髓束 reticulospinal tract
13. 脊髓顶盖束 spinotectal tract
14. 顶盖脊髓束 tectospinal tract
15. 橄榄脊髓束 olivospinal tract
16. 前角外侧核群 lateral nucleus group of anterior horn
17. 前庭脊髓束 vestibulospinal tract
18. 前角内侧核群 medial nucleus group of anterior horn
19. 内侧纵束 medial longitudinal fasciculus
20. 皮质脊髓前束 anterior corticospinal tract
21. 中央管 central canal
22. 白质前索 anterior funiculus of white matter
23. 灰质前角 anterior horn of grey matter
24. 白质外侧索 lateral funiculus of white matter
25. 灰质后角 posterior horn of grey matter
26. 白质后索 posterior funiculus of white matter

图 9-2 脊髓横切面 Transverse sections through spinal cord

A. 颈段，左侧半为髓鞘染色，右侧半为主要核团和纤维束示意图
At a cervical level, left half shows myelin stain, right half for schematic overview
of main nucleus groups and fiber tracts

B. 颈段，髓鞘染色 At a cervical level, myelin stain   C. 胸段，髓鞘染色 At a thoracic level, myelin stain

D. 腰段，髓鞘染色 At a lumbar level, myelin stain   E. 骶段，髓鞘染色 At a sacral level, myelin stain

221

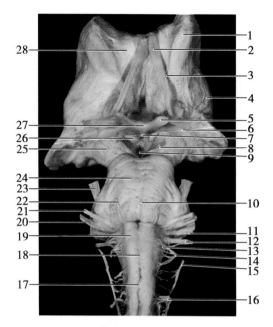

图 9-3 脑干(前面观)
Brain stem(anterior view)

1. 辐射冠 corona radiata
2. 嗅球 olfactory bulb
3. 嗅束 olfactory tract
4. 豆状核 lentiform nucleus
5. 视神经(Ⅱ) optic nerve(Ⅱ)
6. 视束 optic tract
7. 漏斗 infundibulum
8. 动眼神经(Ⅲ) oculomotor nerve(Ⅲ)
9. 脚间窝 interpeduncular fossa
10. 基底沟 basilar sulcus
11. 舌咽神经(Ⅸ) glossopharyngeal nerve(Ⅸ)
12. 迷走神经(Ⅹ) vagus nerve(Ⅹ)
13. 橄榄 olive
14. 舌下神经(Ⅻ) hypoglossal nerve(Ⅻ)
15. 副神经(Ⅺ) accessory nerve(Ⅺ)
16. 第一颈神经 first cervical spinal nerve
17. 锥体交叉 pyramidal decussation
18. 前正中裂 anterior median fissure
19. 锥体 pyramid
20. 前庭蜗神经(Ⅷ) vestibulocochlear nerve(Ⅷ)
21. 面神经(Ⅶ) facial nerve(Ⅶ)
22. 展神经(Ⅵ) abducens nerve(Ⅵ)
23. 三叉神经(Ⅴ) trigeminal nerve(Ⅴ)
24. 脑桥 pons
25. 大脑脚 crus cerebri
26. 乳头体 mamillary body
27. 视交叉 optic chiasma
28. 尾状核 caudate nucleus

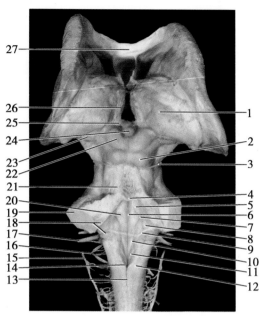

图 9-4 脑干(后面观)
Brain stem(posterior view)

1. 背侧丘脑 dorsal thalamus
2. 下丘 inferior colliculus
3. 滑车神经(Ⅳ) trochlear nerve(Ⅳ)
4. 前髓帆 anterior medullary velum
5. 内侧隆起 medial eminence
6. 正中沟 median sulcus
7. 界沟 sulcus limitans
8. 前庭区 vestibular area
9. 髓纹 striae medullares
10. 舌下神经三角 hypoglossal trigone
11. 迷走神经三角 vagal trigone
12. 楔束结节 cuneate tubercle
13. 后正中沟 posterior median sulcus
14. 薄束结节 gracile tubercle
15. 副神经(Ⅺ) accessory nerve(Ⅺ)
16. 舌下神经(Ⅻ) hypoglossal nerve(Ⅻ)
17. 迷走神经(Ⅹ) vagus nerve(Ⅹ)
18. 小脑下脚 inferior cerebellar peduncle
19. 小脑中脚 middle cerebellar peduncle
20. 面丘 facial colliculus
21. 小脑上脚 superior cerebellar peduncle
22. 上丘 superior colliculus
23. 内侧膝状体 medial geniculate body
24. 松果体 pineal body
25. 缰三角 habenular trigone
26. 丘脑髓纹 thalamic medulary stria
27. 胼胝体 corpus callosum

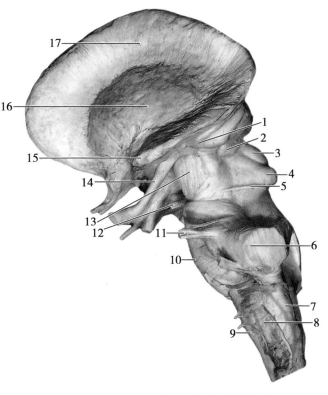

图 9-5　脑干（左侧面观）
Brain stem（left lateral view）

1. 外侧膝状体 lateral geniculate body
2. 内侧膝状体 medial geniculate body
3. 上丘 superior colliculus
4. 下丘 inferior colliculus
5. 滑车神经（Ⅳ）trochlear nerve（Ⅳ）
6. 小脑中脚 middle cerebellar peduncle
7. 小脑下脚 inferior cerebellar peduncle
8. 橄榄 olive
9. 锥体 pyramid
10. 脑桥 pons
11. 三叉神经（Ⅴ）trigeminal nerve（Ⅴ）
12. 动眼神经（Ⅲ）oculomotor nerve（Ⅲ）
13. 大脑脚 crus cerebri
14. 视束 optic tract
15. 杏仁体 amygdala
16. 豆状核 lentiform nucleus
17. 辐射冠 corona radiata

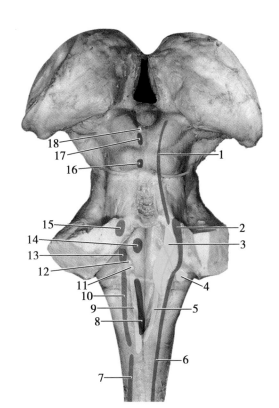

图 9-6　脑干（后面观，图解示意
脑神经核的位置）
Brain stem（posterior view, schematic overview
of locations of cranial nerve nuclei）

1. 三叉神经中脑核 trigeminal mesencephalic nucleus
2. 三叉神经脑桥核 trigeminal pontine
   nucleus
3. 前庭神经核 vestibular nuclei
4. 蜗神经核 cochlear nucleus
5. 孤束核 nucleus of solitary tract
6. 三叉神经脊束核 trigeminal spinal nucleus
7. 副神经脊核 spinal nucleus of
   accessory nerve
8. 舌下神经核 hypoglossal nucleus
9. 迷走神经背核 dorsal vagal nucleus
10. 疑核 nucleus ambiguus
11. 下泌涎核 inferior salivatory nucleus
12. 上泌涎核 superior salivatory nucleus
13. 面神经核 facial motor nucleus
14. 展神经核 abducens nucleus
15. 三叉神经运动核 trigeminal
    motor nucleus
16. 滑车神经核 trochlear nucleus
17. 动眼神经核 oculomotor nucleus
18. 动眼神经副核 accessory
    oculomotor nucleus

223

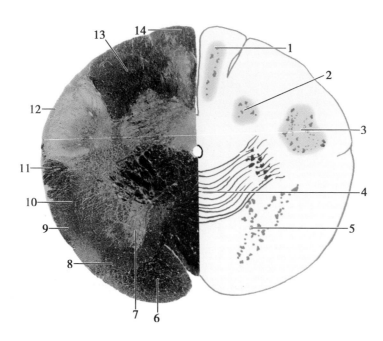

1. 薄束核 nucleus gracilis
2. 楔束核 nucleus cuneatus
3. 三叉神经脊束核 trigeminal spinal nucleus
4. 锥体交叉 pyramidal decussation
5. 副神经脊核 spinal nucleus of accessory nerve
6. 锥体束 pyramidal tract
7. 灰质前角 anterior horn of grey matter
8. 前庭脊髓束 vestibulospinal tract
9. 脊髓小脑前束 anterior spinocerebellar tract
10. 脊髓丘脑束 spinothalamic tract
11. 脊髓小脑后束 posterior spinocerebellar tract
12. 三叉神经脊束 spinal tract of trigeminal nerve
13. 楔束 fasciculus cuneatus
14. 薄束 fasciculus gracilis

图 9-7 延髓横切面(经锥体交叉)
Transverse section through medulla oblongata(at level of pyramidal decussation)
左侧半为髓鞘染色,右侧半为主要核团和纤维束示意图
Left half shows myelin stain,right half for schematic overview of main nucleus groups and fiber tracts

1. 薄束核 nucleus gracilis
2. 楔束核 nucleus cuneatus
3. 三叉神经脊束核 trigeminal spinal nucleus
4. 疑核 nucleus ambiguus
5. 舌下神经核 hypoglossal nucleus
6. 内侧丘系交叉 decussation of medial lemniscus
7. 内侧副橄榄核 medial accessory olivary nucleus
8. 锥体束 pyramidal tract
9. 脊髓小脑前束 anterior spinocerebellar tract
10. 脊髓丘脑束 spinothalamic tract
11. 脊髓小脑后束 posterior spinocerebellar tract
12. 内弓状纤维 internal arcuate fibers
13. 三叉神经脊束 spinal tract of trigeminal nerve
14. 楔束 fasciculus cuneatus
15. 薄束 fasciculus gracilis

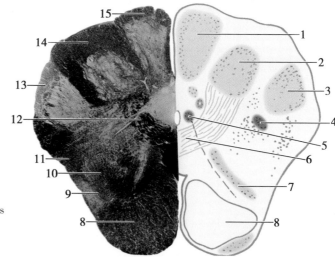

图 9-8 延髓横切面(经内侧丘系交叉)
Transverse section through medulla oblongata(at level of decussation of medial lemniscus)
左侧半为髓鞘染色,右侧半为主要核团和纤维束示意图
Left half shows myelin stain,right half for schematic overview of main nucleus groups and fiber tracts

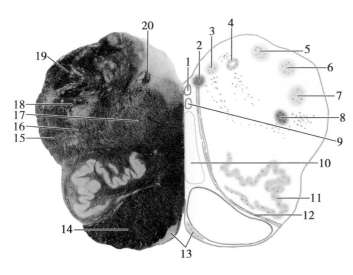

1. 内侧纵束 medial longitudinal fasciculus
2. 舌下神经核 hypoglossal nucleus
3. 迷走神经背核 dorsal vagal nucleus
4. 孤束核 nucleus tractus solitarius
5. 前庭神经下核 inferior vestibular nucleus
6. 楔束副核 accessory cuneate nucleus
7. 三叉神经脊束核 trigeminal spinal nucleus
8. 疑核 nucleus ambiguus
9. 顶盖脊髓束 tectospinal tract
10. 内侧丘系 medial lemniscus
11. 下橄榄核 inferior olivary nucleus
12. 舌下神经纤维 fibers of hypoglossal nerve
13. 弓状核 arcuate nucleus
14. 锥体束 pyramidal tract
15. 脊髓小脑前束 anterior spinocerebellar tract
16. 脊髓丘脑束 spinothalamic tract
17. 网状结构 reticular formation
18. 三叉神经脊束 spinal tract of trigeminal nerve
19. 小脑下脚 inferior cerebellar peduncle
20. 孤束 solitary tract

图 9-9　延髓横切面（经下橄榄核中部）
Transverse section through medulla oblongata（at level of middle part of inferior olive nucleus）
左侧半为髓鞘染色，右侧半为主要核团和纤维束示意图
Left half shows myelin stain，right half for schematic overview of main nucleus groups and fiber tracts

1. 内侧纵束 medial longitudinal fasciculus
2. 舌下神经核 hypoglossal nucleus
3. 前庭神经内侧核 medial vestibular nucleus
4. 孤束核 nucleus of solitary tract
5. 前庭神经下核 inferior vestibular nucleus
6. 蜗背侧核 dorsal cochlear nucleus
7. 顶盖脊髓束 tectospinal tract
8. 蜗腹侧核 ventral cochlear nucleus
9. 三叉神经脊束核 trigeminal spinal nucleus
10. 疑核 nucleus ambiguus
11. 内侧丘系 medial lemniscus
12. 下橄榄核 inferior olivary nucleus
13. 锥体束 pyramidal tract
14. 脊髓丘脑束 spinothalamic tract
15. 三叉神经脊束 spinal tract of trigeminal nerve
16. 小脑下脚 inferior cerebellar peduncle
17. 网状结构 reticular formation

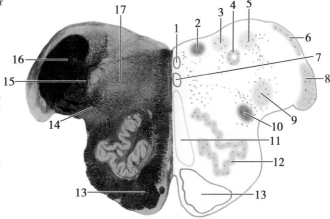

图 9-10　延髓横切面（经蜗神经核）
Transverse section through medulla oblongata（at level of cochlear nuclei）
左侧半为髓鞘染色，右侧半为主要核团和纤维束示意图
Left half shows myelin stain，right half for schematic overview of main nucleus groups and fiber tracts

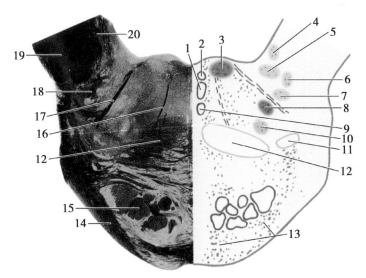

图 9-11　脑桥横切面(经面丘)
Transverse section through pons(at level of facial colliculus)
左侧半为髓鞘染色,右侧半为主要核团和纤维束示意图
Left half shows myelin stain,right half for schematic overview of main nucleus groups and fiber tracts

1. 内侧纵束 medial longitudinal tract
2. 面神经膝 genu of facial nerve
3. 展神经核 abducens nucleus
4. 前庭神经上核 superior vestibular nucleus
5. 前庭神经内侧核 medial vestibular nucleus
6. 前庭神经外侧核 lateral vestibular nucleus
7. 三叉神经脊束核 trigeminal spinal nucleus
8. 面神经核 facial motor nucleus
9. 顶盖脊髓束 tectospinal tract
10. 上橄榄核 superior olivary nucleus
11. 外侧丘系 lateral lemniscus
12. 内侧丘系和斜方体 medial lemniscus and trapezoid body
13. 脑桥核 pontine nuclei
14. 脑桥横纤维 transverse fibers of pons
15. 锥体束 pyramidal tract
16. 展神经纤维 fibers of abducens nerve
17. 面神经纤维 fibers of facial nerve
18. 三叉神经脊束 spinal tract of trigeminal nerve
19. 小脑中脚 middle cerebellar peduncle
20. 小脑上脚 superior cerebellar peduncle

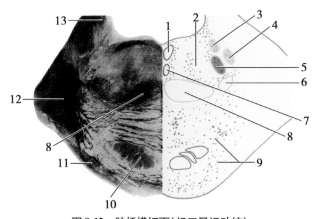

图 9-12　脑桥横切面(经三叉运动核)
Transverse section through pons(at level of trigeminal motor nucleus)
左侧半为髓鞘染色,右侧半为主要核团和纤维束示意图
Left half shows myelin stain,right half for schematic overview of main nucleus groups and fiber tracts

1. 内侧纵束 medial longitudinal fasciculus
2. 网状结构 reticular formation
3. 三叉神经中脑核 trigeminal mesencephalic nucleus
4. 三叉神经脑桥核 trigeminal pontine nucleus
5. 三叉神经运动核 trigeminal motor nucleus
6. 外侧丘系 lateral lemniscus
7. 顶盖脊髓束 tectospinal tract
8. 内侧丘系 medial lemniscus
9. 脑桥核 pontine nuclei
10. 锥体束 pyramidal tract
11. 脑桥横纤维 transverse fibers of pons
12. 小脑中脚 middle cerebellar peduncle
13. 小脑上脚 superior cerebellar peduncle

226

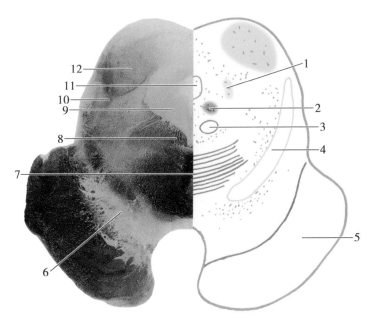

1. 三叉神经中脑核 trigeminal mesencephalic nucleus
2. 滑车神经核 trochlear nucleus
3. 内侧纵束 medial longitudinal fasciculus
4. 内侧丘系 medial lemniscus
5. 大脑脚 crus cerebri
6. 黑质 substantia nigra
7. 小脑上脚交叉 decussation of superior cerebellar peduncle
8. 顶盖脊髓束 tectospinal tract
9. 中央灰质 central gray matter
10. 外侧丘系 lateral lemniscus
11. 大脑水管 cerebral aqueduct
12. 下丘核 nucleus of inferior colliculus

图 9-13 中脑横切面(经下丘)
Transverse section through midbrain(at level of inferior colliculus)
左侧半为髓鞘染色,右侧半为主要核团和纤维束示意图
Left half shows myelin stain,right half for schematic overview of main nucleus groups and fiber tracts

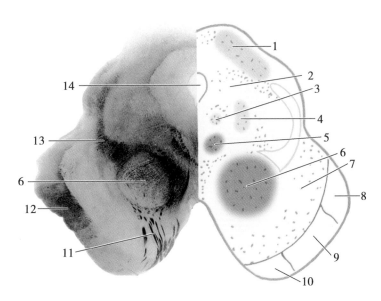

图 9-14 中脑横切面(经上丘)
Transverse section through midbrain(at level of superior colliculus)
左侧半为髓鞘染色,右侧半为主要核团和纤维束示意图
Left half shows myelin stain,right half for schematic overview of main nucleus groups and fiber tracts

1. 上丘灰质层 gray matter layer of superior colliculus
2. 中央灰质 central gray matter
3. 动眼神经副核 accessory oculomotor nucleus
4. 三叉神经中脑核 trigeminal mesencephalic nucleus
5. 动眼神经核 oculomotor nucleus
6. 红核 red nucleus
7. 黑质 substantia nigra
8. 顶颞桥束 parietotemporopontine tract
9. 锥体束 pyramidal tract
10. 额桥束 frontopontine tract
11. 动眼神经(Ⅲ)纤维 fibers of oculomotor nerve(Ⅲ)
12. 大脑脚 crus cerebri
13. 内侧丘系 medial lemniscus
14. 大脑水管 cerebral aqueduct

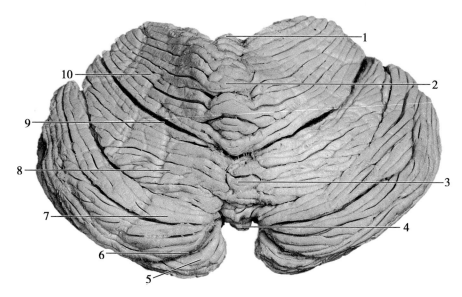

图 9-15　小脑（上面观）
Cerebellum（superior view）

1. 中央小叶 central lobule
2. 山顶 culmen
3. 山坡 declive
4. 蚓叶 folium of vermis
5. 下半月小叶 inferior semilunar lobule

6. 水平裂 horizontal fissure
7. 上半月小叶 superior semilunar lobule
8. 后方形小叶部 posterior quadrangular lobule
9. 原裂 primary fissure
10. 前方形小叶 anterior quadrangular lobule

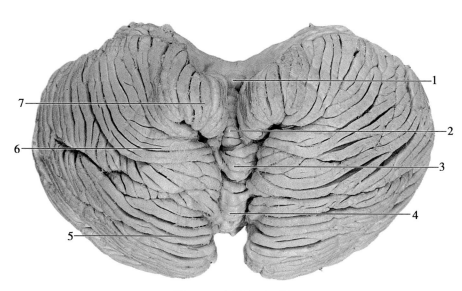

图 9-16　小脑（下面观）
Cerebellum（inferior view）

1. 小结 nodule
2. 蚓垂 uvula of vermis
3. 蚓锥体 pyramid of vermis
4. 蚓结节 tuber of vermis

5. 下半月小叶 inferior semilunar lobule
6. 二腹小叶 biventral lobule
7. 小脑扁桃体 tonsil of cerebellum

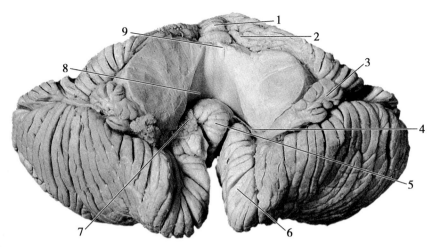

图 9-17　小脑(前面观)
Cerebellum(anterior view)

1. 中央小叶 central lobule
2. 中央小叶翼 ala of central lobule
3. 绒球 flocculus
4. 绒球脚 peduncle of flocculus
5. 小结 nodule
6. 小脑扁桃体 tonsil of cerebellum
7. 第四脑室脉络丛 choroid plexus of fourth ventricle
8. 第四脑室 fourth ventricle
9. 上髓帆 superior medullary velum

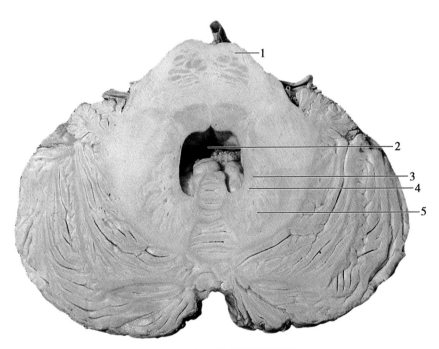

图 9-18　小脑横断面(下面观)
Transverse section through cerebellum(inferior view)

1. 脑桥 pons
2. 第四脑室 fourth ventricle
3. 球状核 globose nucleus
4. 栓状核 emboliform nucleus
5. 齿状核 dentate nucleus

229

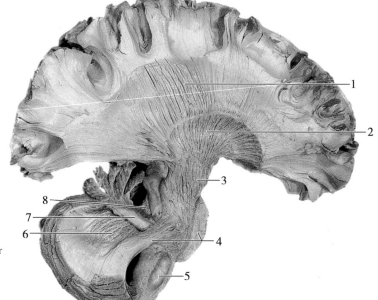

1. 辐射冠 corona radiata
2. 内囊 internal capsule
3. 锥体束 pyramidal tract
4. 小脑中脚 middle cerebellar peduncle
5. 橄榄 olive
6. 齿状核 dentate nucleus
7. 小脑下脚 inferior cerebellar peduncle
8. 小脑上脚 superior cerebellar peduncle

图 9-19　小脑脚及锥体束(右外侧面观)
Cerebellar peduncles and pyramidal tract (right lateral view)

1. 尾状核 caudate nucleus
2. 豆状核 lentiform nucleus
3. 杏仁体 amygdala
4. 视束 optic tract
5. 视神经 optic nerve
6. 漏斗 infundibulum
7. 大脑脚 crus cerebri
8. 脑桥 pons
9. 三叉神经(Ⅴ) trigeminal nerve(Ⅴ)
10. 前庭蜗神经(Ⅷ) vestibulocochlear nerve(Ⅷ)
11. 小脑中脚 middle cerebellar peduncle
12. 齿状核 dentate nucleus
13. 小脑上脚 superior cerebellar peduncle
14. 下丘 inferior colliculus
15. 内侧膝状体 medial geniculate body
16. 上丘 superior colliculus
17. 外侧膝状体 lateral geniculate body

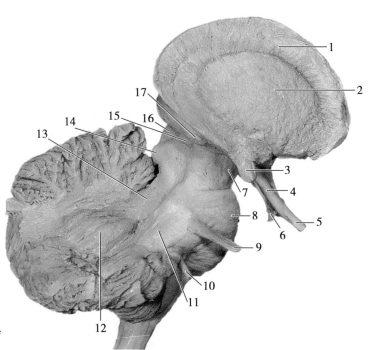

图 9-20　基底节和脑干(右外侧面观)
Basal ganglia and brain stem (right lateral view)

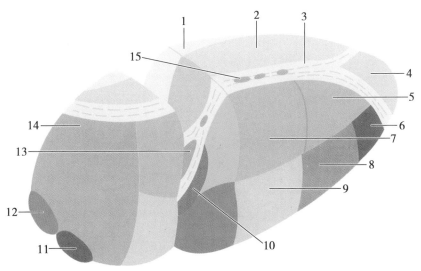

图 9-21　丘脑核团模式图
Diagram of thalamic nuclei

1. 中线核群 midline nuclei
2. 内侧背核 mediodorsal nucleus
3. 内髓板 internal medullary lamina
4. 前核群 anterior nuclei
5. 背外侧核群 dorsal lateral nuclei
6. 腹前核 ventral anterior nucleus
7. 外侧后核 lateral posterior nucleus
8. 腹外侧核 ventral lateral nucleus

9. 腹后外侧核 ventral posterolateral nucleus
10. 腹后内侧核 ventral posteromedial nucleus
11. 外侧膝状体 lateral geniculate body
12. 内侧膝状体 medial geniculate body
13. 中央中核 centromedian nucleus
14. 丘脑枕 pulvinar
15. 板内核群 intralaminar nuclei

1. 室间孔 interventricular foramen
2. 丘脑间黏合 interthalamic adhesion
3. 背内侧核 dorsomedial nucleus
4. 下丘脑沟 hypothalamic sulcus
5. 后核 posterior nucleus
6. 腹内侧核 ventromedial nucleus
7. 乳头体 mamillary body
8. 弓状核（漏斗核）arcuate nucleus（infundibular nucleus）
9. 视上核 supraoptic nucleus
10. 视交叉 optic chiasma
11. 视前内侧核 medial preoptic nucleus
12. 视前外侧核 lateral preoptic nucleus
13. 前核 anterior nucleus
14. 室旁核 paraventricular nucleus

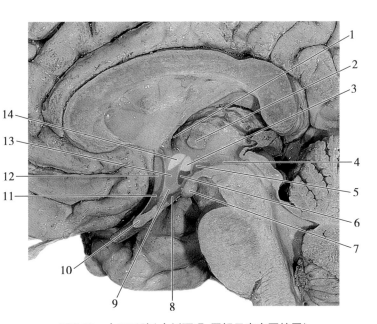

图 9-22　右下丘脑（内侧面观，图解示意主要核团）
Right hypothalamus（medial view，schematic overview location of main nuclei）

231

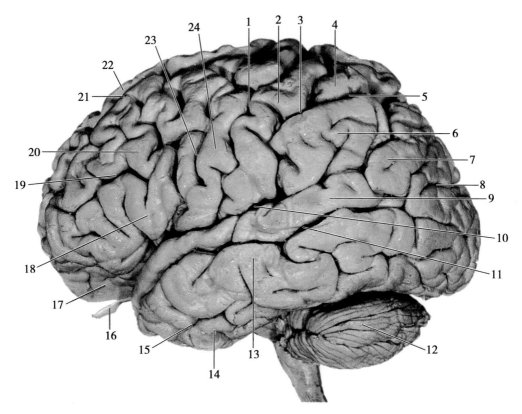

图 9-23　脑（左外侧面观）
Brain（left lateral view）

1. 中央沟 central sulcus	13. 颞中回 middle temporal gyrus
2. 中央后回 postcentral gyrus	14. 颞下回 inferior temporal gyrus
3. 中央后沟 postcentral sulcus	15. 颞下沟 inferior temporal sulcus
4. 顶上小叶 superior parietal lobule	16. 嗅球 olfactory bulb
5. 顶内沟 intraparietal sulcus	17. 眶回 orbital gyri
6. 缘上回 supramarginal gyrus	18. 额下回 inferior frontal gyrus
7. 角回 angular gyrus	19. 额下沟 inferior frontal sulcus
8. 顶枕沟 parietooccipital sulcus	20. 额中回 middle frontal gyrus
9. 颞上回 superior temporal gyrus	21. 额上沟 superior frontal sulcus
10. 外侧裂 lateral fissure	22. 额上回 superior frontal gyrus
11. 颞上沟 superior temporal sulcus	23. 中央前沟 precentral sulcus
12. 小脑 cerebellum	24. 中央前回 precentral gyrus

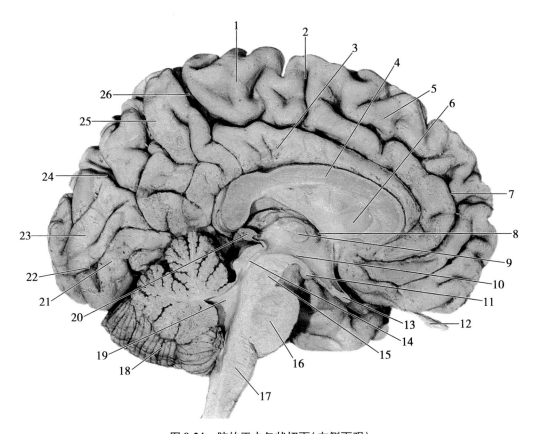

图 9-24　脑的正中矢状切面 (左侧面观)
Median sagittal section through brain (left lateral view)

1. 中央旁小叶 paracentral lobule
2. 中央旁沟 paracentral sulcus
3. 扣带回 cingulate gyrus
4. 胼胝体 corpus callosum
5. 额上回 superior frontal gyrus
6. 透明隔 septum pellucidum
7. 扣带沟 cingulate sulcus
8. 室间孔 interventricular foramen
9. 丘脑间黏合 interthalamic adhesion
10. 下丘脑沟 hypothalamic sulcus
11. 乳头体 mamillary body
12. 嗅球 olfactory bulb
13. 视交叉 optic chiasma
14. 大脑水管 cerebral aqueduct
15. 中脑 midbrain
16. 脑桥 pons
17. 延髓 medulla oblongata
18. 小脑 cerebellum
19. 第四脑室 fourth ventricle
20. 松果体 pineal body
21. 舌回 lingual gyrus
22. 距状沟 calcarine sulcus
23. 楔叶 cuneus
24. 顶枕沟 parietooccipital sulcus
25. 楔前叶 precuneus
26. 缘支 marginal ramus

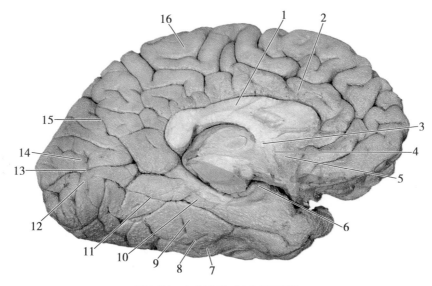

图 9-25　左大脑半球（内侧面观）
Left cerebral hemisphere（medial view）

1. 胼胝体 corpus callosum	9. 枕颞内侧回 medial occipitotemporal gyrus
2. 扣带回 cingulate gyrus	10. 海马旁回 parahippocampal gyrus
3. 前连合 anterior commissure	11. 侧副沟 collateral sulcus
4. 终板旁回 paraterminal gyrus	12. 舌回 lingual gyrus
5. 胼胝体下区 subcallosal area	13. 距状沟 calcarine sulcus
6. 钩 uncus	14. 楔叶 cuneus
7. 枕颞外侧回 lateral occipitotemporal gyrus	15. 顶枕沟 parietooccipital sulcus
8. 枕颞沟 occipitotemporal sulcus	16. 中央旁小叶 paracentral lobule

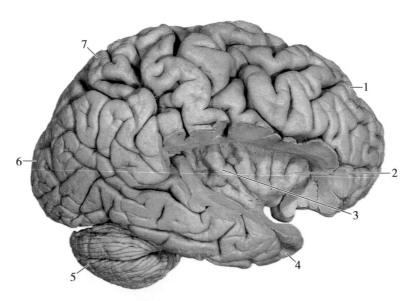

图 9-26　右脑岛（外侧面观）
Right insula（lateral view）

1. 额叶 frontal lobe	5. 小脑 cerebellum
2. 岛短回 short gyri of insula	6. 枕叶 occipital lobe
3. 岛长回 long gyrus of insula	7. 顶叶 parietal lobe
4. 颞叶 temporal lobe	

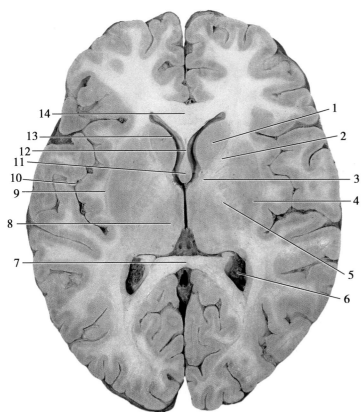

1. 尾状核头 head of caudate nucleus
2. 内囊前肢 anterior limb of internal capsule
3. 内囊膝 genu of internal capsule
4. 豆状核 lentiform nucleus
5. 内囊后肢 posterior limb of internal capsule
6. 侧脑室后角 posterior horn of lateral ventricle
7. 胼胝体压部 splenium of corpus callosum
8. 丘脑 thalamus
9. 屏状核 claustrum
10. 脑岛 insula
11. 穹窿柱 column of fornix
12. 透明隔 septum pellucidum
13. 侧脑室前角 anterior horn of lateral ventricle
14. 胼胝体膝 genu of corpus callosum

图 9-27　脑的水平切面(上面观)
Transverse section through brain(superior view)

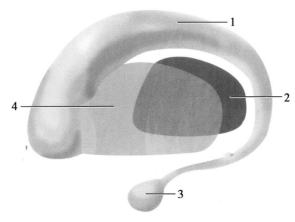

图 9-28　左基底节(外侧观)
Left basal ganglia(lateral view)

1. 尾状核 caudate nucleus
2. 背侧丘脑 dorsal thalamus
3. 杏仁体 amygdala
4. 豆状核 lentiform nucleus

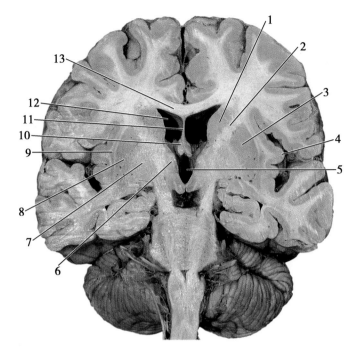

图 9-29 脑的冠状切面 (前面观)
Coronal section through brain
(anterior view)

1. 尾状核 caudate nucleus
2. 内囊 internal capsule
3. 豆状核 lentiform nucleus
4. 脑岛 insula
5. 第三脑室 third ventricle
6. 丘脑 thalamus
7. 苍白球 globus pallidus
8. 壳 putamen
9. 屏状核 claustrum
10. 穹窿 fornix
11. 透明隔 septum pellucidum
12. 侧脑室 lateral ventricle
13. 胼胝体 corpus callosum

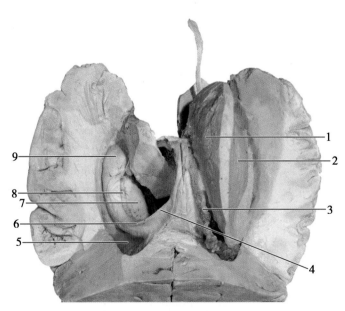

图 9-30 侧脑室下角 (上面观)
Inferior horn of lateral ventricle (superior view)

1. 尾状核 caudate nucleus
2. 豆状核 lentiform nucleus
3. 侧脑室脉络丛 choroid plexus of lateral ventricle
4. 穹窿脚 crus of fornix
5. 侧副三角 collateral trigone
6. 海马伞 fimbria of hippocampus
7. 海马旁回 parahippocampal gyrus
8. 齿状回 dentate gyrus
9. 海马 hippocampus

236

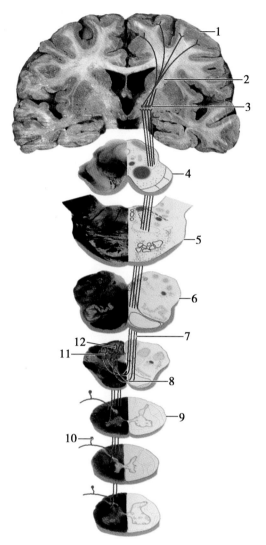

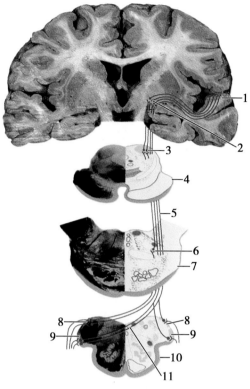

图 9-31 本体感觉传导道示意图
**Schematic overview of pathway for
proprioception**

1. 中央后回 postcentral gyrus
2. 内囊 internal capsule
3. 腹后外侧核 ventral posterolateral nucleus
4. 中脑 midbrain
5. 脑桥 pons
6. 延髓 medulla oblongata
7. 内侧丘系 medial lemniscus
8. 内侧丘系交叉 decussation of medial lemniscus
9. 脊髓 spinal cord
10. 脊神经节 spinal ganglion
11. 楔束核 nucleus cuneatus
12. 薄束核 nucleus gracilis

图 9-32 听觉传导道示意图
Schematic overview of auditory pathway

1. 颞横回 transverse temporal gyrus
2. 内侧膝状体 medial geniculate body
3. 下丘核 nucleus of inferior colliculus
4. 中脑 midbrain
5. 外侧丘系 lateral lemniscus
6. 上橄榄核 superior olivary nucleus
7. 脑桥 pons
8. 蜗背侧核 dorsal cochlear nucleus
9. 蜗腹侧核 ventral cochlear nucleus
10. 延髓 medulla oblongata
11. 斜方体 trapezoid body

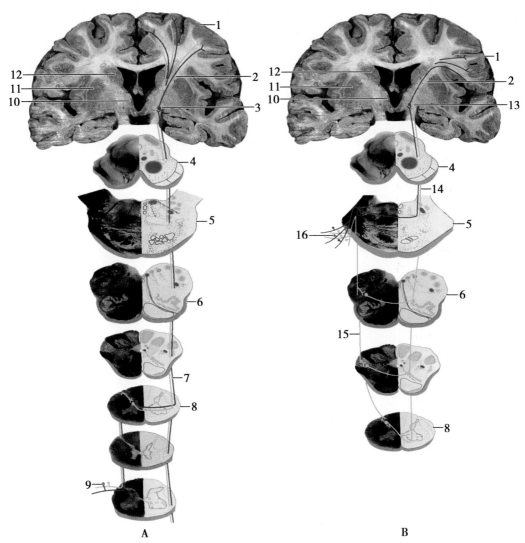

A　　　　　　　　　　　　　　　　B

图 9-33　痛觉、温觉传导道示意图
Schematic overview of pathway for pain and temperature

A. 脊丘系 Spinal lemniscus　B. 三叉丘系 Trigeminal lemniscus

1. 中央后回 postcentral gyrus
2. 内囊 internal capsule
3. 腹后外侧核 ventral posterolateral nucleus
4. 中脑 midbrain
5. 脑桥 pons
6. 延髓 medulla oblongata
7. 脊髓丘脑束 spinothalamic tract
8. 脊髓 spinal cord

9. 脊神经节 spinal ganglion
10. 背侧丘脑 dorsal thalamus
11. 豆状核 lentiform nucleus
12. 尾状核 caudate nucleus
13. 腹后内侧核 ventral posteromedial nucleus
14. 三叉丘系 trigeminal lemniscus
15. 三叉神经脊束 spinal tract of trigeminal nerve
16. 三叉神经节 trigeminal ganglion

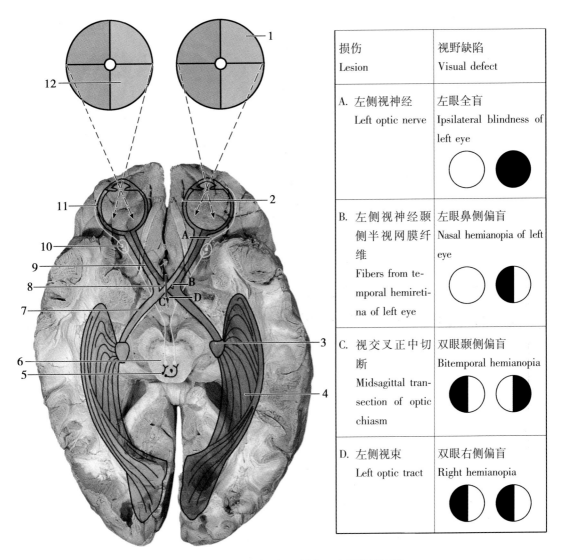

损伤 Lesion	视野缺陷 Visual defect
A. 左侧视神经 Left optic nerve	左眼全盲 Ipsilateral blindness of left eye
B. 左侧视神经颞侧半视网膜纤维 Fibers from temporal hemiretina of left eye	左眼鼻侧偏盲 Nasal hemianopia of left eye
C. 视交叉正中切断 Midsagittal transection of optic chiasm	双眼颞侧偏盲 Bitemporal hemianopia
D. 左侧视束 Left optic tract	双眼右侧偏盲 Right hemianopia

图 9-34　视觉传导道及视野缺损示意图（下面观）
Schematic overview of visual pathway and visual defects associated with various
lesions along visual pathway（inferior view）

1. 颞侧视野 temporal visual field
2. 鼻侧半视网膜 nasal half of retina
3. 外侧膝状体 lateral geniculate body
4. 视辐射 optic radiation
5. 顶盖前区 pretectal area
6. 动眼神经副核 accessory oculomotor nucleus
7. 视束 optic tract
8. 视交叉 optic chiasma
9. 视神经（Ⅱ）optic nerve（Ⅱ）
10. 睫状神经节 ciliary ganglion
11. 颞侧半视网膜 temporal half of retina
12. 鼻侧视野 nasal visual field

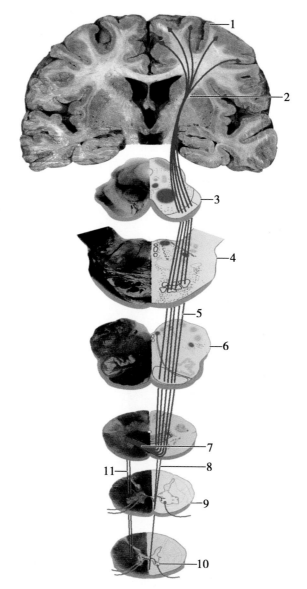

图 9-35 锥体系(皮质脊髓束)示意图
Schematic overview of pyramidal system(corticospinal tracts)

1. 中央前回 precentral gyrus
2. 内囊 internal capsule
3. 中脑 midbrain
4. 脑桥 pons
5. 皮质脊髓束 corticospinal tract
6. 延髓 medulla oblongata
7. 锥体交叉 pyramidal decussation
8. 皮质脊髓前束 anterior corticospinal tract
9. 脊髓 spinal cord
10. 灰质前角 anterior horn of grey matter
11. 皮质脊髓侧束 lateral corticospinal tract

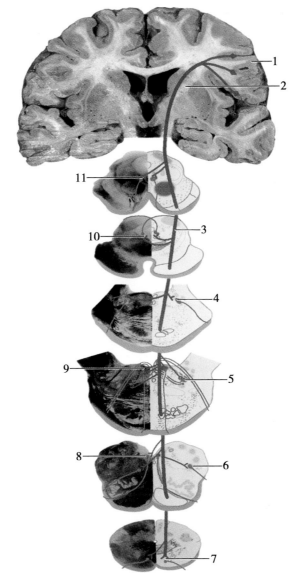

图 9-36　锥体系（皮质核束）示意图
Schematic overview of pyramidal system（corticonuclear tract）

1. 中央前回 precentral gyrus
2. 内囊 internal capsule
3. 皮质核束 corticonuclear tract
4. 三叉神经运动核 motor nucleus of trigeminal nerve
5. 面神经核 facial motor nucleus
6. 疑核 nucleus ambiguus
7. 副神经脊核 spinal nucleus of accessory nerve
8. 舌下神经核 hypoglossal nucleus
9. 展神经核 abducens nucleus
10. 滑车神经核 trochlear nucleus
11. 动眼神经核 oculomotor nucleus

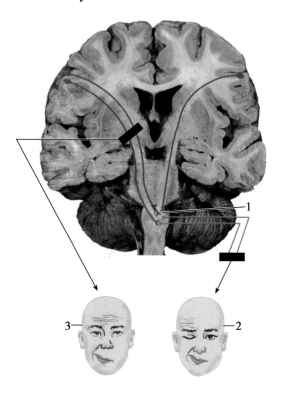

图 9-37　面神经瘫示意图
Schematic overview of facial nerve paralysis

1. 面神经核 facial motor nucleus
2. 面神经核下瘫 infranuclear paralysis
3. 面神经核上瘫 supranuclear paralysis

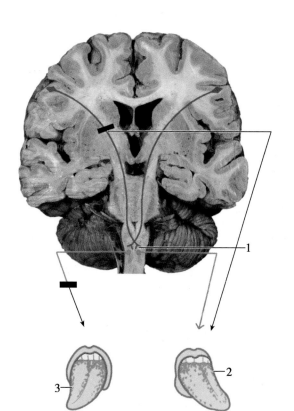

图 9-38　舌下神经瘫示意图
Schematic overview of hypoglossal paralysis

1. 舌下神经核 hypoglossal nucleus
2. 舌下神经核上瘫 supranuclear paralysis
3. 舌下神经核下瘫 infranuclear paralysis

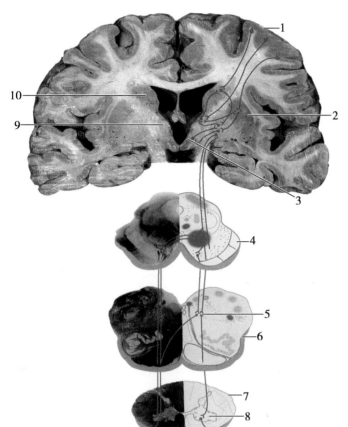

图 9-39　锥体外系（纹状体苍白球联系）示意图
Schematic overview of extrapyramidal system（striopallidal connection）
1. 大脑皮质 cerebral cortex
2. 豆状核 lentiform nucleus
3. 底丘脑核 subthalamic nucleus
4. 中脑 midbrain
5. 网状结构 reticular formation
6. 延髓 medulla oblongata
7. 脊髓 spinal cord
8. 灰质前角 anterior horn of grey matter
9. 丘脑 thalamus
10. 尾状核 caudate nucleus

图 9-40　锥体外系（皮质脑桥小脑联系）
Schematic overview of extrapyramidal system（corticopontocerebellar connection）
1. 丘脑 thalamus
2. 豆状核 lentiform nucleus
3. 齿状丘脑束 dentatothalamic tract
4. 齿状核 dentate nucleus
5. 脑桥小脑束 pontocerebellar tract
6. 脊髓小脑后束 posterior spino-cerebellar tract
7. 红核脊髓束 rubrospinal tract
8. 齿状红核束 dentatorubral tract
9. 脑桥核 pontine nuclei
10. 红核 red nucleus

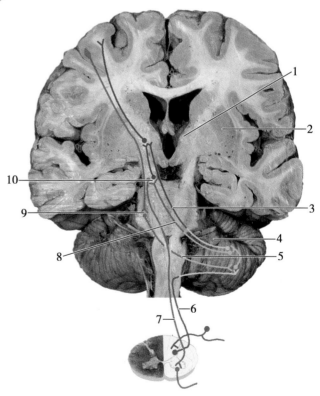

243

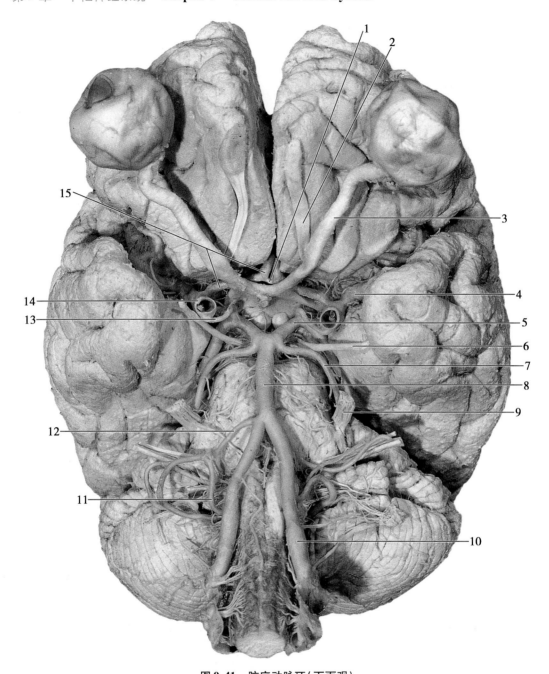

图 9-41 脑底动脉环(下面观)
Circulus arteriosus at base of brain(inferior view)

1. 前交通动脉 anterior communicating artery
2. 嗅束 olfactory tract
3. 视神经(Ⅱ) optic nerve(Ⅱ)
4. 大脑中动脉 middle cerebral artery
5. 大脑后动脉 posterior cerebral artery
6. 动眼神经(Ⅲ) oculomotor nerve(Ⅲ)
7. 小脑上动脉 superior cerebellar artery
8. 基底动脉 basilar artery
9. 三叉神经(Ⅴ) trigeminal nerve(Ⅴ)
10. 椎动脉 vertebral artery
11. 小脑后下动脉 posterior inferior cerebellar artery
12. 小脑前下动脉 anterior inferior cerebellar artery
13. 后交通动脉 posterior communicating artery
14. 颈内动脉 internal carotid artery
15. 大脑前动脉 anterior cerebral artery

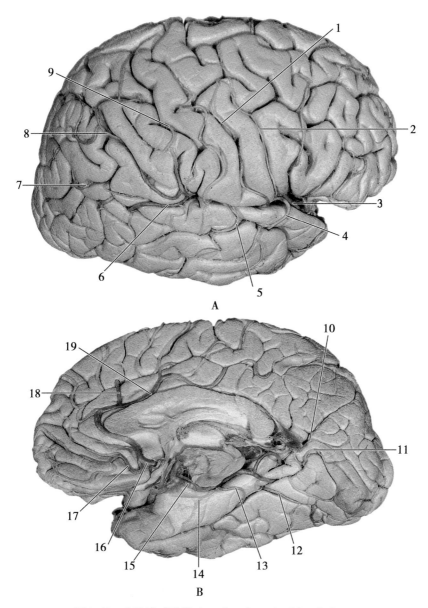

图 9-42　大脑半球动脉 Arteries of cerebral hemisphere
A. 外侧面 Lateral surface　B. 内侧面 Medial surface

1. 中央沟动脉 central artery
2. 中央前沟动脉 precentral artery
3. 大脑中动脉 middle cerebral artery
4. 颞前动脉 anterior temporal artery
5. 颞中动脉 middle temporal artery
6. 颞后动脉 posterior temporal artery
7. 角回动脉 angular artery
8. 顶后动脉 posterior parietal artery
9. 中央后沟动脉 postcentral artery
10. 顶枕动脉 parietooccipital artery

11. 距状沟动脉 calcarine artery
12. 颞后支 posterior temporal branch
13. 颞中间支 intermediate temporal branch
14. 颞前支 anterior temporal branch
15. 大脑后动脉 posterior cerebral artery
16. 大脑前动脉 anterior cerebral artery
17. 额极动脉 frontopolar artery
18. 胼胝体缘动脉 callosomarginal artery
19. 胼胝体周动脉 pericallosal artery

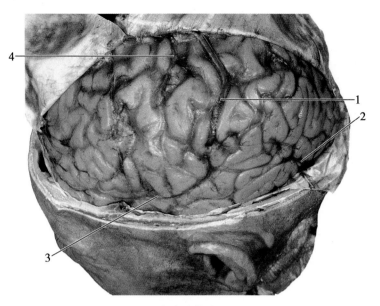

图 9-43　大脑半球的静脉（左外侧面观）
Veins of cerebral hemisphere（left lateral view）

1. 上吻合静脉 superior anastomotic vein
2. 下吻合静脉 inferior anastomotic vein
3. 大脑浅中静脉 superficial middle cerebral vein
4. 大脑上静脉 superior cerebral vein

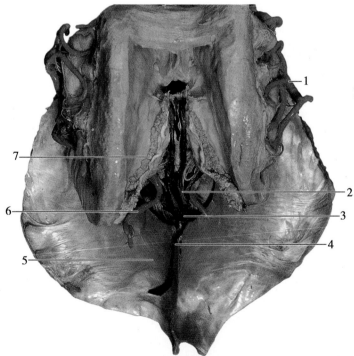

图 9-44　大脑深静脉（上面观）
Deep cerebral veins（superior view）

1. 大脑中动脉 middle cerebral artery
2. 大脑内静脉 internal cerebral vein
3. 大脑大静脉 great cerebral vein
4. 直窦 straight sinus
5. 小脑幕 tentorium of cerebellum
6. 大脑后动脉 posterior cerebral artery
7. 侧脑室脉络丛 choroid plexus of lateral ventricle

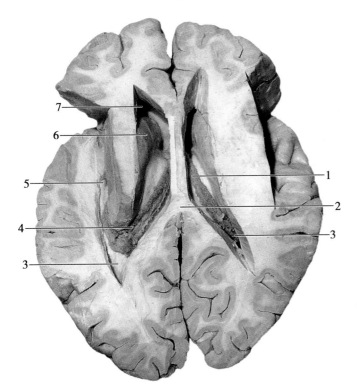

图 9-45　侧脑室（上面观）
Lateral ventricle（superior view）

1. 侧脑室中央部 central part of lateral ventricle
2. 胼胝体压部 splenium of corpus callosum
3. 侧脑室后角 posterior horn of lateral ventricle
4. 侧脑室脉络丛 choroid plexus of lateral ventricle
5. 海马 hippocampus
6. 尾状核头 head of caudate nucleus
7. 侧脑室前角 anterior horn of lateral ventricle

1. 视神经 optic nerve
2. 视交叉 optic chiasma
3. 颈内动脉 internal carotid artery
4. 动眼神经 oculomotor nerve
5. 幕切迹 tentorial incisure
6. 小脑幕 tentorium of cerebellum
7. 横窦 transverse sinus
8. 窦汇 confluence of sinuses
9. 直窦 straight sinus
10. 上矢状窦 superior sagittal sinus
11. 大脑镰 falx cerebri

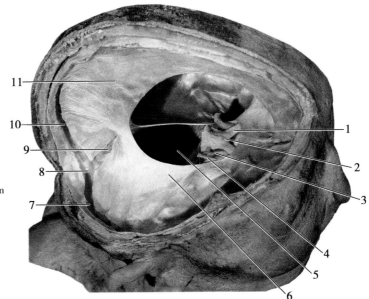

图 9-46　硬脑膜及硬脑膜静脉窦（右外侧面观）
Cerebral dura mater and dural venous sinuses（right lateral view）

247

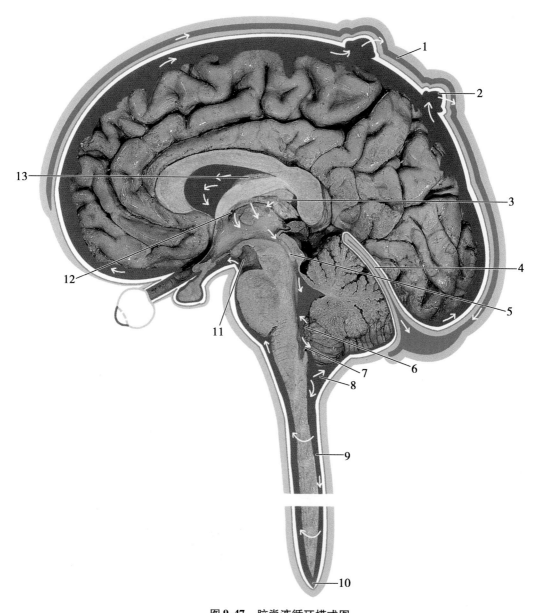

图 9-47　脑脊液循环模式图
Diagram of cerebrospinal fluid circulation

1. 上矢状窦 superior sagittal sinus
2. 蛛网膜粒 arachnoid granulation
3. 第三脑室脉络丛 choroid plexus of third ventricle
4. 直窦 straight sinus
5. 大脑水管 cerebral aqueduct
6. 第四脑室脉络丛 choroid plexus of fourth ventricle
7. 第四脑室正中孔 median aperture of fourth ventricle

8. 小脑延髓池 cerebellomedullary cistern
9. 蛛网膜下腔 subarachnoid space
10. 终池 terminal cistern
11. 脚间池 interpeduncular cistern
12. 室间孔 interventricular foramen
13. 侧脑室脉络丛 choroid plexus of lateral ventricle

索 引
Index

G

H

K

P

R

X

Y